Policy Futures for UK Health

Edited by

Zoë Slote Morris

Nuffield Fellow in Health Policy
Judge Business School
University of Cambridge

Linda Rosenstrøm Chang

Research Assistant
Policy Futures for UK Health project
Judge Business School
University of Cambridge

Sandra Dawson

Director
Judge Business School
University of Cambridge

and

Pam Garside

Senior Associate
Judge Business School
University of Cambridge

Foreword by

Denis Pereira Gray

Chairman of the Trustees

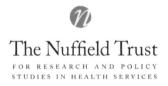

The Nuffield Trust

FOR RESEARCH AND POLICY
STUDIES IN HEALTH SERVICES

Radcliffe Publishing
Oxford • Seattle

Radcliffe Publishing Ltd
18 Marcham Road
Abingdon
Oxon OX14 1AA
United Kingdom

www.radcliffe-oxford.com
Electronic catalogue and worldwide online ordering facility.

British Library Cataloguing in Publication Data

A catalogue record for this book is available from the British Library.

ISBN 1 84619 003 7

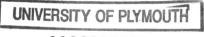
Typeset by Advance Typesetting Ltd, Oxford
Printed and bound by TJ International Ltd, Padstow, Cornwall

Contents

Foreword

There is tremendous interest in the future of the health of people and their health-care and, for health professionals and planners, professionally so.

Overall, the health of the British population is steadily improving; life expectation continues to rise and outcomes, for most diseases, slowly improve. In the future, more is to be expected of individual patients in doing more both to preserve health and in participating in their own healthcare. Healthcare will become more complicated, more expensive, and will be provided by a greater number and variety of carers.

Many of the drivers of healthcare in the future are well known, such as increasing technology, the ageing of the population, increased expectation of consumers and, the commonest accompanying consequence in western countries, a rising proportion of government budgets spent on health. But why is this and what other factors will be important? What are the likely ethical and legal circumstances in which such changes will occur?

Quite apart from the most likely trends, this book does not shirk the big questions like: Who will govern? Who will do the caring, and what will it all cost? Strikingly, the 'burden of health' is described, highlighting the wide range of costs and consequences which arise from better health.

Separate chapters on all these and other topics provide detailed facts and figures which inform and underpin the conclusions drawn. Many of these chapters, and indeed the book as a whole, should prove useful as reference and source material for organisations planning discussions on their own future.

Of course, no-one can ever precisely foresee the future, but good information and analysis does make a great deal possible. The Trust is encouraged by the justification of the conclusions of its first publication in this series (Dargie *et al.*, 2000), which influence Government policy.

This work can be taken into account with other work from the Trust on the current quality of healthcare such as Leatherman and Sutherland (2003, 2005) who authoritatively describe much of the current position in healthcare in the UK.

The Nuffield Trust is an independent charity, free to publish on its own account. It has concentrated on studying the future for several years and this book is the second in a series, with a third publication still to come. This is the biggest and longest running research project on the future of health and healthcare in the UK. The Trustees hope it will help to inform all those interested and to stimulate informed discussions on the many issues that arise, and the Trust welcomes comments.

The Trustees thank the broad based advisory group whose members contributed many ideas. Zoë Slote Morris has been the Nuffield Trust Fellow, working with Linda Rosenstrøm Chang and Pam Garside at the Judge Business School of the University of Cambridge, under the direction of Dame Sandra Dawson, and the Trust is most grateful to them.

Sir Denis Pereira Gray OBE, HonDSc, FRCP, FRCGP, FMedSci
Chairman of the Trustees
October 2005

References

Dargie C *et al.* (2000) *Policy Futures for UK Health*. The Stationery Office, London for The Nuffield Trust and the University of Cambridge.

Leatherman S and Sutherland K (2003) *Quest for Quality*. The Stationery Office, London for The Nuffield Trust.

Leatherman S and Sutherland K (2005) *The Quest for Quality in the NHS: a chartbook on quality of care in the UK*. Radcliffe Publishing, Oxford for The Nuffield Trust.

A Nuffield Trust perspective

The health of an individual depends on a wide range of factors, including lifestyle, environment, heredity and the quality of medical care.

For the past 60 years, The Nuffield Trust has concerned itself with the many issues that have a significant bearing on health and healthcare in the UK in general and the ways in which these issues have an impact on individual well-being.

This report marks an important contribution to the health debate. It is designed to stimulate policy makers and other stakeholders to think afresh about the relationships that link government, health providers, carers and the increasingly knowledgeable – and assertive – citizens they serve.

There is no single solution to improving healthcare and health status in 21st century Britain. That is why this report represents the diverse points of view of several experts in their fields.

However, from this diversity several themes emerge. Taken together, they clearly indicate that this country needs a new health settlement for the new century. This settlement, which will probably need to be based on a new Health of the People Act, should effectively redefine the relationships between government and people and between the NHS and patients. While preserving the commitment to maintain a NHS free at the point of delivery, it should be more explicit about the responsibilities of individuals in maintaining their own health.

A new health act would be a major step by any standards. But then so was the creation of the NHS over half a century ago. It was a measure that reflected society as it was and effectively transformed healthcare in the UK. But life in 21st century Britain is virtually unrecognisable from that of those post-war years. The UK has changed and new legislation should reflect the way we live now.

The impact of ageing

One of the most significant themes emphasised in this report is the advancing age of the UK population and the impact that already has – and will continue to have – on health and healthcare.

A boy born in the UK today can expect to live for 75 years or more. But it is likely that he will be ill for six of those years. A girl can look forward to more than 80 years of life; but she will live a tenth of that time with at least a degree of infirmity. Who will look after these people?

Since 2001 there has been a distinct population shift, with more people over 60 than there are under 16. The implications of this are clear. What this report refers to as the nation's 'dependency ratio' is increasing. In other words, a diminishing workforce will have to support a growing dependent population who are living longer than their parents and grandparents thanks to advances in medical science, the wider availability of medical care and improvements in public health.

Even now, there are about six million carers in Britain – most of them looking after elderly parents or relatives and often spending more than 50 hours a week doing so. Of these carers, about a third are themselves over 60. As the pension crisis delays the age of retirement, such carers will be in even shorter supply.

Another issue compounds the problem of an ageing population. The longer people live, the more susceptible they are to a number of diseases and chronic conditions including cancer, arthritis and rheumatism. Currently half a million people suffer from Alzheimer's disease in the UK. By 2020, that figure is expected to double. Clearly, increasing longevity is going to impose an ever greater burden on individuals and society.

By 2025, as much as half the population could be suffering from chronic disease. One consequence of this problem is likely to be the blurring of the boundaries between the types of care that people will require in future: health and social; formal and informal. Of course, this situation could present opportunities as well as concerns. With appropriate management, there might be a significant shift in focus from secondary care to primary care; from prevention to cure; to health rather than healthcare.

However, if this is to happen another issue must be addressed as well: growing health inequalities and inequities.

Health for all?

An unmistakable and unedifying message that this report reiterates is the linkage between health and economic and social determinants: How much you own, your employment (or lack of it) and where you live tend to influence the state of your health.

To some extent, this has probably always been true. But the growing disparity between rich and poor in the past 20 years has exacerbated this ethical and social dilemma to a degree that becomes morally unacceptable.

Government initiatives to help tackle this problem have been in place for some years, including the Social Exclusion Unit in England which was specifically established to deal with those root causes of inequalities most associated with poorer health.

As the report indicates, the need for such efforts seems to be more immediate now than ever in recent history, with some of the greatest threats to health most closely associated with poverty. For example, the UK has the highest rate of overweight and obese people in the European Union. In a decade the proportion of obese men has risen from 13% to 21% for men and from 15% to 24% for women. Even more alarmingly, the proportion of obese children rose from just over 12% to 15.6%. If this trend continues, at least one third of adults, one fifth of boys and one third of girls will be obese by 2020.

Obesity is statistically associated with poverty. So are smoking and the abuse of alcohol and drugs.

The results of these conditions are all too apparent in the prevalence and consequences of cancer, mental illness, accidents, obesity, diabetes, heart disease and strokes. Mortality rates are 70% higher in the most deprived areas than in the most affluent. Or, to put it bluntly, the poorer you are, the more likely you are to die early.

Such inequalities are not only unnecessary and avoidable, they could also be considered violations of the Human Rights Act 1998. The question is how best to eliminate or at least reduce such reprehensible disparities. Unfortunately, as the report shows, this problem could be compounded by the increasing significance of another approach to improving health efficiencies for the wider population: self-care.

A prescription for self-reliance

To what extent can individuals be expected to take responsibility for their own health?

Current health promotion policies advocate a partnership between citizens and health professionals. This philosophy has a number of implications. Among them is the potential for significant savings. Full engagement, in which citizens follow expert advice to keep themselves healthy, inevitably results in less costly healthcare provision. Other costs, however, can rise.

To be effective, self-care must be taught, learned, maintained and sustained. It must be 'co-created' by the individual and the system. These imperatives call for a significant commitment to programmes that not only encompass health but also IT proficiency to enable the internet access on which much self-care now depends. Therefore, the concept of self-care calls for changes across education and lifestyle as well as healthcare systems. In both, there will have to be increased emphasis on a broad range of topics. In addition to personal health, these include effective parenting and childcare, fitness and nutrition.

In time, self-care could extend to the management of chronic illnesses – freeing up vast resources now handled by the public sector. This is already happening in the treatment of asthma, using well-defined clinical protocols while simultaneously taking some of the strain off the NHS. Similar independence is available to those with high cholesterol levels, who can now arrange to receive their simvastatin prescriptions through direct deals with their pharmacists.

Appealing as the concept of self-care might be, it is questionable whether improved health is, in itself, a sufficient incentive to involve individuals to the extent required. Will people need further inducements to take greater responsibility for their own care? This could raise the costs of what otherwise seems a cost-effective alternative to traditional healthcare.

Self-care has built-in limitations as well. The concept takes as self-evident that individuals must prefer to take care of themselves. As the report notes, this assumption is not always valid. Nor is everyone equally capable of administering self-care. For whatever reasons, some can never manage it. Others lose the ability to administer self-care with increasing age or infirmity. To cope with such circumstances, there has to be a network of support mechanisms, including provision of the means to assess a person's self-care potential.

Again, technology can play a role in this. In fact, technology – in all its manifestations – is probably the single most important factor in the transformation of healthcare in the UK.

The impact of technology

In the field of healthcare, technology is an unequivocally good thing. It prolongs lives and improves the quality of those lives. It informs and empowers. It triggers further innovation. But it will almost inevitably increase costs and raises some complex ethical issues. For these reasons, there is no obvious 'right' policy path to take in the alliance between technology and healthcare in the 21st century. Instead, choices will be made on the basis of selecting 'conflicting goods': economic development versus cost-containment or public funding versus private profit.

That said, there are tensions in the application of technological breakthroughs to healthcare requirements. Perhaps this is due to the fact that technology development is largely driven by commercial sector investment. As a result, it is not always directly or initially appropriate to the needs of the healthcare sector and the people who work in it. This conflict could probably be resolved through government incentives for the development of appropriate healthcare technologies – in the field of primary care perhaps.

The ethical questions raised by some technologies are more difficult to address. For example, developments in genetics and the use of human tissue will have to be resolved with formal policy responses and appropriate legislation drafted within an ethical framework.

Equally important is the notion of privacy in a world that increasingly seeks the full transparency offered by breakthroughs in information technology. Again, the report notes, this is a matter for government, working to a structured and well-designed public education strategy.

Above all, technology is creating empowerment through information. Self-care is a case in point. But self-care can also engender self-confidence to the point at which patients will question – or even challenge – the opinions and actions of the professionals looking after them.

This is already altering traditional relationships throughout the care chain, affecting doctors, nurses, technicians, support staff and of course the patients themselves.

The era of the expert patient

Patient passivity is becoming a thing of the past.

In the 21st century, individuals define themselves as consumers. Whether they are buying fashion, holidays or their morning coffee, they increasingly demand and revel in the widest possible range of choices. Increasingly, they take the same approach to managing their health and selecting their healthcare options.

A consumer is driven by expectations. In the healthcare sector, these expectations include a reasonably long life lived with as much comfort and freedom from pain as possible. Expectations also encompass the type of care they receive to deliver these objectives. The broad array of complementary and alternative therapies available has widened choice even further.

It is up to healthcare professionals to recognise such expectations and, when necessary, manage them. As the report notes, growing awareness about healthcare choices tends to raise expectations. In healthcare these cannot always be met. The result can be disappointment. For example, recent research suggests that the proportion of people satisfied with hospital services has fallen to just over 50%.

One explanation for this might be the chronic shortage of healthcare professionals in the UK. The nation's 500 000 nurses and 130 000 doctors are already thinly stretched. Rising patient demands and expectations will make the situation even less tenable. One solution highlighted in the report is the transformation of care by shifting roles and professional boundaries.

More teamwork and less hierarchy among healthcare professionals will, however, require the development of different skills and attitudes. Fortunately, this is already occurring. Nurse practitioners are a prime example. Patients like them because they can spend more time in consultation than doctors and prescribe medication as necessary without delay. Management likes them because they are less costly. And nurse practitioners themselves tend to enjoy the greater degree of job satisfaction that goes with enhanced autonomy and responsibility.

Bringing it all together

It is one thing to highlight emerging themes in 21st century UK healthcare. It is even more of a challenge to find the links between themes that could result in more effective, 'joined-up' policy. *Policy Futures for UK Health 2005* does both.

Looking ahead to 2020, the report focuses on five cross-cutting themes or policy areas that are woven through the document as a whole. These are:

- the determinants of health
- equity and equality
- individual and community expectations of healthcare and health
- science, technology and industrial policy
- information, evaluation and benchmarking.

Policy Futures addresses each of these in detail. This discussion urges policy makers to broaden their thinking along these lines to encompass the wider picture. In this way, the UK will be better placed to tackle the vital issues that remain for health in Britain in the period to 2020.

Foremost among these issues is the need for a greater emphasis on individual health and well-being as a basic entitlement in the 21st century, and not merely part of a greater public good. To do this, we will need to review and restate the values that underpin current health policy. This is bound to have major implications for responsibilities and funding.

The importance of the individual notwithstanding, UK health policy has to be viewed within broader social and global contexts as well.

The economic context of healthcare is equally significant. With the current budget for the NHS alone running at close to £70 billion, democratic, clinical and corporate governance must be the centre of every policy agenda. That is why the report calls for a review of the purpose and scope of public and patient involvement in health policy.

It is down to the government to play a leading strategic role in all of this, helping to build a more rational and planned system than the one currently in place. Ideally, government could share this stewardship with an independent body immune to election cycles and better able to work across sectors.

Meanwhile, as the report shows, the UK is suffering a genuine crisis in care, with funds, workers and facilities in short supply. Those who are most affected by these resource constraints are those who are least able to cope.

Policy Futures provides a realistic assessment of the current state of healthcare in the UK, raises the need for further research in several vital areas and offers helpful insights on how best to shape a future that affects us all.

Everyone involved – authors, consultation participants, members of the Policy and Evaluation Advisory Group – deserve the sincere thanks of The Nuffield Trust. In particular, credit is due to the team at the Judge Institute.

Thanks to their efforts, we are considerably closer to a viable vision for a healthier nation.

Kim Beazor
Chief Operating Officer
The Nuffield Trust
October 2005

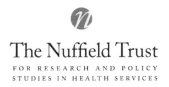

The Nuffield Trust

FOR RESEARCH AND POLICY
STUDIES IN HEALTH SERVICES

The Nuffield Trust is one of the leading independent health policy charitable trusts in the UK. It was established as the Nuffield Provincial Hospitals Trust in 1940 by Viscount Nuffield (William Morris), the founder of Morris Motors. In 1998 the Trustees agreed that the official name of the Trust should more fully reflect the Trust's purposes and, in consultation with the Charity Commission, adopted the name The Nuffield Trust for Research and Policy Studies in Health Services, retaining 'The Nuffield Trust' as its working name.

The Nuffield Trust mission is to promote independent analysis and informed debate on UK healthcare policy. The Nuffield Trust's purpose is to communicate evidence and encourage an exchange around developed or developing knowledge in order to illuminate recognised and emerging issues.

It achieves this through the following principal activities.

- Bringing together a wide national and international network of people involved in UK healthcare through a series of meetings, workshops and seminars.
- Commissioning research through its publications and grants programme to inform policy debate.
- Encouraging interdisciplinary exchange between clinicians, legislators, academics, healthcare professionals and management, policymakers, industrialists and consumer groups.
- Supporting evidence-based health policy and practice.
- Sharing its knowledge in the home countries and internationally through partnerships and alliances.

To find out more please refer to our website or contact:

The Nuffield Trust
59 New Cavendish St
London
W1G 7LP
Website: www.nuffieldtrust.org.uk
Email: mail@nuffieldtrust.org.uk
Tel: +44 (0)20 7631 8458
Fax: +44 (0)20 7631 8451

Charity number: 209201

List of Trustees

Patron

About the editors

Sandra Dawson BA (Hons), MA (Cantab) is Director of Judge Business School, University of Cambridge, where she also holds the KPMG Professorship of Management Studies. She is also Master of Sidney Sussex College, Cambridge. She writes and consults on organisational behaviour, health management, innovation and technology transfer and is author of numerous articles and four books.

Pam Garside BSc (Hons), MHA has her own management consultancy, Newhealth, specialising in organisational strategy and development in healthcare in the UK and internationally. She is a Senior Associate at Judge Business School, University of Cambridge, where she is also Co-Director of the Cambridge International Health Leadership Programme.

Linda Rosenstrøm Chang BSc, BA, MA is a Research Assistant on the Policy Futures for UK Health project based at Judge Business School, University of Cambridge. Previously she has worked on refugee employment and integration, urban regeneration in London and human rights advocacy in the Commonwealth.

Zoë Slote Morris BSc (Econ) Hons, PG Dip, PhD is currently the Nuffield Fellow responsible for the Policy Futures for UK Health project at Judge Business School, University of Cambridge. Her main research interests relate to evaluation and public policy. Previous work has focused on dental and medical education and drug treatment services. She has also published on young people and social capital.

List of contributors

Raj Bhopal CBE, MPH, MD, FRCPE is the Alexander Bruce and John Usher Professor of Public Health and Head of the Division on Community Health Services, Public Health Services Section, University of Edinburgh, Scotland.

Don E Detmer MD, MA is President and Chief Executive Officer of the American Medical Informatics Association, a trustee of The Nuffield Trust, a member of the Institute of Medicine and fellow of AAAS, ACMI and ACS. He has chaired the Board on Health Care Services (IOM), the National Committee on Vital and Health Statistics and the Board of Regents, National Library of Medicine.

Tony Hope MA, PhD, MBBCh, FRCPsych, MFPH is Professor of Medical Ethics at the University of Oxford, Honorary Consultant Psychiatrist and Director of Ethox. He has carried out research in basic neuroscience and Alzheimer's disease. His books include *Oxford Handbook of Clinical Medicine* (Editions one to four), *Manage Your Mind, Medical Ethics and Law: the core curriculum* and *Medical Ethics: a very short introduction.*

Alison Kitson RN, BSc (Hons), PhD, FRCN is Executive Director of Nursing at the Royal College of Nursing (RCN). As part of the RCN's team, she is responsible for leading on the organisation's professional nursing agenda and helping it deliver its mission to represent nurses and nursing, promoting excellence in practice and shaping health policies.

Graham Lister BSc, MSc, PhD is a Senior Associate of Judge Business School, University of Cambridge. He is an international expert on health policy, leadership and management. He was healthcare consultancy partner of Coopers and Lybrand, Chair of the College of Health, served on the National Institute for Clinical Excellence Partners Council and Buckinghamshire Health Authority and has worked with WHO, World Bank, IMF and DH.

Domhnall MacAuley MD, FRCGP, FFPHMI, FFSEM, FISM, DPH, DRCOG, DSM, Dip Sports Med is a general practitioner in Belfast and an assistant editor at the *BMJ*. He is honorary professor in the Faculty of Life Science at the University of Ulster and is former Professor of Primary Health Care Research. He has written or edited six books and over 200 academic publications.

Sheila McLean LLB, MLitt, PhD, LLD, FRSE, FRCGP, FRCP, FRSA is Director at the Institute of Law and Ethics in Medicine, University of Glasgow and is an expert in medical law. She is a Fellow of the Royal Society of Edinburgh and an Honorary Fellow of the Royal College of General Practitioners and the Royal College of Physicians of Edinburgh. She holds honorary doctorates from the Universities of Abertay and Edinburgh.

Alison Petch BA (Hons), MA, DipSW, PhD is Nuffield Trust Professor of Community Care Public Health and Health Policy, University of Glasgow and currently heads a research group, originally funded by The Nuffield Trust, which focuses on the study of community care policy and practice in a multidisciplinary and multi-agency context. She has a particular interest in patterns of support for older people and for people with mental health problems.

Ray Robinson BA, MSc (Econ) is Professor of Health Policy at LSE Health and Social Care, London School of Economics. Previously, he has also worked at the University of Southampton, the King's Fund Institute and HM Treasury. His work at LSE is concerned with various aspects of health finance, economics and management.

Suzanne Wait MA, PhD is Nuffield Trust Research Fellow at Judge Business School, University of Cambridge. Her research at Cambridge has focused on benchmarking and public involvement. She has a PhD in Health Policy from University of Strasbourg and a Masters of Public Health from Columbia University. She is also Director of Research at the International Longevity Centre-UK. Other research interests include age discrimination in healthcare and comparative European health policy.

Ron Zimmern MA, MB, FRCP, FFPHM was appointed Director of the Cambridge Genetics Knowledge Park in Cambridge in April 2002. He is also the Director of the Public Health Genetics Unit (from June 1997) and the Institute of Public Health at the University of Cambridge (from January 2003).

List of abbreviations

A number of abbreviations, which may be unfamiliar, appear regularly in this book, and include the following.

AIDS	Acquired immune deficiency syndrome
ASH	Action on Smoking and Health
BMA	British Medical Association
BMJ	British Medical Journal
CAM	Complementary and alternative medicine
CHAI	Commission for Healthcare Audit and Inspection
CHD	Coronary heart disease
DALYs	Disability-adjusted life years
DCMS	Department of Culture, Media and Sport
DfES	Department for Education and Skills
DH	Department of Health
DWP	Department of Work and Pensions
EBM	Evidence-based medicine
ECJ	European Court of Justice
EEA	European Economic Area
EFSA	European Food and Safety Authority
EU	European Union
FCO	Foreign and Commonwealth Office
GDP	Gross domestic product
GNP	Gross national product
GP	General practitioner (medical doctor)
HIV	Human immunodeficiency virus
HPA	Health Protection Agency
HSJ	Health Service Journal
HTA	Health Technology Assessment
ICT	Information and communication technology
IT	Information technology
LIFT	Local Improvement Finance Trust
MMR	Measles, mumps and rubella
NHS	National Health Service
NICE	National Institute for Clinical Excellence
NIHCE	National Institute for Health and Clinical Excellence
NMC	Nursing and Midwifery Council
NPfIT	National Programme for Information Technology
NSF	National Service Framework
OECD	Organisation for Economic Co-operation and Development

PACTS	Parliamentary Advisory Council for Transport Safety
PBR	Payment by result
PCO	Primary Care Organisation
PCT	Primary Care Trust
PEAG	Policy and Evaluation Advisory Group
PFI	Private Finance Initiative
PSSRU	Personal Social Services Research Unit
R&D	Research and Development
RPBWP	Research for Patient Benefit Working Party
SHA	Strategic Health Authority
TB	Tuberculosis
TC	Treatment centre
TSO	The Stationery Office
UK	United Kingdom
UKCC	United Kingdom Central Council for Nursing (now the NMC)
UN	United Nations
WHO	World Health Organization

Acknowledgements

There are many people to whom we are grateful for their contribution to the *Policy Futures* project. We would especially like to thank John Wyn Owen, former Secretary of The Nuffield Trust. He led the project from its inception in 1998 and chaired the Policy and Evaluation Advisory Group (PEAG).

PEAG was appointed by The Nuffield Trust to guide the project and its members include: Professor Raj Bhopal, Alexander Bruce and John Usher Professor of Public Health, University of Edinburgh; Professor Sir Les Borysiewicz, Deputy Rector, Imperial College; Professor Sir Ara Darzi, Faculty of Medicine, Imperial College; Professor Dame Sandra Dawson, Director of Judge Business School, University of Cambridge; Professor Don E Detmer, President and Chief Executive Officer, American Medical Informatics Association, Professor Emeritus & Professor of Medical Education at the University of Virginia, Senior Associate at Judge Business School, University of Cambridge; Pam Garside, Senior Associate of The Nuffield Trust and Judge Business School; Professor Sir Denis Pereira Gray, Chair of The Nuffield Trust; Dr Scott L Greer, Assistant Professor of Health Management and Policy at the University of Michigan School of Public Health and member of the Constitution Unit, University College London; Professor Tony Hope, Director of The Ethox Centre and Professor of Medical Ethics, University of Oxford; Professor Alison Kitson, Executive Director of Nursing at the Royal College of Nursing; Janet Lewis-Jones; Dr Graham Lister, Senior Associate of Judge Business School; Professor Domhnall MacAuley, Hillhead Family Practice and honorary professor in the Faculty of Life Science at the University of Ulster; Professor Sheila McLean, Director of the Institute of Law and Ethics in Medicine, University of Glasgow; Alison Petch, Nuffield Trust Professor of Community Care, University of Glasgow; Ray Robinson, Professor of Health Policy at LSE Health and Social Care, London School of Economics and Political Science; and Dr Ron Zimmern, Director of the Cambridge Genetics Knowledge Park, the Public Health Genetics Unit and the Institute of Public Health, University of Cambridge. We are grateful to all of the members for their commitment, time and thoughtful contributions.

Colleagues at The Nuffield Trust played an important role in facilitating the organisation and administration of the project. Particular recognition is owed to Kim Beazor, Olivia Roberts, and to Helena Scott for support throughout the publishing stage. We are also appreciative to members of Judge Business School who gave their time and energy. Dr Suzanne Wait enthusiastically devoted her time to the Environmental Scan and Marie-Ann Kyne-Lilley provided continuity from the first phase of the project. Stephan Luis updated the Environmental Scan and Kiare Ladner provided editorial support.

Finally, we would like to thank all of those who participated with enthusiasm and commitment in our various consultation processes.

Zoë Slote Morris
Linda Rosenstrøm Chang
Sandra Dawson
Pam Garside
October 2005

Introduction

Sandra Dawson, Zoë Slote Morris and Linda Rosenstrøm Chang

The Policy Futures for UK Health project, funded by the Nuffield Trust, identifies issues likely to be relevant to health and wellbeing over the next 15 years. It considers the resulting implications for policy with a threefold purpose to:

- aid policy development by highlighting the more predictable trends in health
- explore the contingent nature of policy and future outcome, such as the way in which different models of regulation might lead to different technological futures
- allow stakeholders an opportunity to plan for policy changes necessary to achieve a preferred future.

This book is the final outcome of the project. It anticipates developments in the health environment up to 2020, evaluates current and planned policy developments using a futures approach, identifies themes which crosscut policy and makes recommendations to government.

The book covers all parts of the UK but divergence in health policy since devolution is not the main focus. Discussion of health and wellbeing is not limited to management of the NHS and other treatment providers, but includes wider determinants of health.

Policy Futures for UK Health 2000

A previous publication, *Policy Futures for UK Health 2000 Report* (Dargie *et al.*, 2000), highlighted three key messages of need:

- to keep a long-term health and wellbeing perspective as a priority across all policy
- to manage and pay for patient and public expectations
- to plan workforce issues in the context of social, economic and technical change.

Underpinning the first report's recommendations was the need for effective installation and use of information technology (IT), as well as better utilisation of data.

Many of the issues raised have been addressed during the period between the first and second reports, for example, the National Programme for IT (NPfIT).

There has also been a sustained increase in the NHS budget since 2002. Although some argue that most of this additional funding is earmarked or squeezed by cost pressures rendering only 2.5 to 3% as uncommitted 'additional' funding (Appleby, 2005), the increase of 7.5% overall marks the largest single increase in NHS funding since its establishment.

There is also debate over the likely impact of the additional funds. The Office of National Statistics (ONS), for example, reports that productivity in England did not grow between 1997 and 2003 (ONS, 2004). As ONS states, however, productivity measures to date do not allow for 'quality changes'. Work is already underway to improve productivity measures, and quality improvements have occurred.

The *Quest for Quality in the NHS* report (Leatherman and Sutherland, 2003) estimates that more than £235 million was spent on quality improvement between 1999 and 2003, and that this brought about improvements in the quality of care across most areas. Furthermore, it concludes that the NHS shows 'capacity to improve' and, with continuing financial support and reform, improvement will continue. Although issues such as poor information and the effect of perverse incentives still need to be addressed, the overall message is positive. Leatherman and Sutherland (2005) published coincidentally with this volume provides further evidence of positive change, together with key areas for remedial action.

A greater focus on health and wellbeing can be discerned (DH, 2004; Wanless, 2004). In the discussion of health service productivity, ONS notes that the positive outcomes it reports – increased life expectancy, reduced infant mortality and reductions in circulatory disease, cancers and respiratory disease – are attributable to factors other than the NHS. Notwithstanding, data show that the NHS is treating more patients, even if it is not yet possible to assess whether increased spending on healthcare has resulted in better health (Panorama, 2005).

Since 2000, there has been considerable reform within health policy, the effect of which has been generally positive. Inevitably, however, difficulties remain and identifying key challenges for the next 15 years is the focus of this book.

Studying futures

Those who believe the future is predictable and largely determined by current forces see futures work as a useful aid to planning. For others, the future is unpredictable and can only be thought of in terms of probabilities and possibilities. Since policy choices are limited and 'the future' is likely to fall between these extremes, futures studies should 'discover or invent, examine, evaluate and propose possible, probable and preferable futures' (Bell, 1997). Futures studies can be seen as being about identifying alternative futures and facilitating 'individuals and groups in formulating, implementing, and re-envisioning their preferred futures' (Dator, 1996).

Method of analysis

While 'there are no facts about the future' (Hicks, 2001), a range of methods can be used to explore the probable, possible and preferable (Coyle, 1997). The environmental scan in this report emerges from an analysis of trend data across a broad range of topics relevant to the wider determinants of health. It is designed to provide a backdrop against which policy needs to be formulated and implemented. Subsequent chapters derive from a review of formal literature and commentary about 'the future'. The intention of looking 15 years into the future is to strike a balance between looking beyond a five-year election cycle but not beyond the imagination or into a future too detached from current policy (Dargie, 2000).

Although the research process has been rigorous, the link between 'evidence' and conclusion, and therefore also recommendations, is subjective. Omissions, misinterpretations and flawed conclusions are perhaps inevitable. To this end, expert opinion has been elicited to bridge gaps in published predictions or to modify expectations. Engagement in wider professional networks and consultation has supplemented the process and responses are reflected in the text (Dator, 1996).

In November 2004, a consultation conference was held in London and attended by 83 people drawn from the Department of Health (DH), NHS trusts, academic institutions, businesses, charities, public organisations and the media. Report topics were presented for further consultation from the Northern Irish perspective at the Medical Society in Belfast in January 2005. The discussions, feedback and commentary that followed these consultations have been incorporated into the report.

Structure of the book

The book consists of three sections. Part 1 looks at the current context. It begins with an 'environmental scan' focusing on the wider determinants of health:

- disease
- society
- environment
- governance
- economics
- industry.

Since one of the tasks of the report is to review and update trends and issues identified in *Policy Futures for UK Health 2000 Report*, each of these sub-sections includes a summary review of relevant current policy that has been announced since 2000.

Also included as context are ethical and legal issues. The implications of these issues – for example in connection with healthcare, health promotion and human rights – are examined in the chapters following the scan and subsequently integrated into the report where relevant.

Part 2 comprises five chapters that explore policy themes raised in the scan in more detail.

- 'Who's going to govern?' addresses the state's relationship with the market, the workforce and the individual engaged in health and healthcare and the issues of responsibility, accountability and public investment.
- 'Who's going to care?' focuses on issues related to supply and demand for care in its broadest sense, including self-care, informal and formal care, in social and health settings.
- 'What will be the burden of health?' looks at diseases and threats to health, across a spectrum ranging from certainty to uncertainty, from chronic disease to bioterrorism.
- 'Where will technology take us?' explores medical technologies and information technology, focusing on factors likely to support or impede their development and diffusion into the health arena by 2020.
- 'What will health cost?' explores issues related to raising funding for health, including challenges for tax-funded health systems in the future, and provides discussion as to how money should be spent.

Each chapter has different authors. The authors were asked to consider issues pertinent to UK health policy within their theme, while taking into account the consultation. Together their work represents a collection of essays intended to promote wider discussion rather than a coherent policy statement. Issues and drivers of change for UK health in 2020 are given consideration, and current and planned policy developments are evaluated. The chapters conclude with a series of recommendations.

Part 3 draws together major themes and provides a short conclusion for the future. As the Policy Futures for UK Health project progressed, the difficulties and limitations of looking at policy themes as discrete entities became increasingly clear. As part of the consultation process, participants were asked to identify themes relevant to more than one policy area. The results of this exercise are presented in Chapter 9 'Where are the linkages for joined-up policy?', which focuses on:

- the determinants of health
- equity and equality
- individual and community expectations of health
- science, technology and industrial policy
- information, evaluation and benchmarking.

The book concludes by identifying the key challenges and opportunities for UK health policy in the future. Figure 1 gives schematic representation to the structure of the book.

References

Appleby J (2005) Data briefing: economic growth and NHS spending. *Health Service Journal.* **23**: 23.

Bell W (1997) *Foundations of Futures Studies.* Transaction Publishers, Somerset, NJ.

Coyle G (1997) The nature and value of futures studies or do futures have a future? *Futures.* **29**(1): 77–93.

Dargie C, Dawson S and Garside P (2000) *Policy Futures for UK Health 2000 Report.* The Nuffield Trust, London.

Dator J (1996) In: R Slaughter (ed.) *The Knowledge Base of Futures Studies.* DDM Media Group, Melbourne.

DH (2004) *Choosing Health: making healthier choices easier. Cmnd 6374.* The Stationery Office, London.

Hicks D (2001) Re-examining the future: the challenge for citizenship education. *Educational Review.* **53**(3): 229–40.

Leatherman S and Sutherland K (2003) *The Quest for Quality in the NHS: a mid-term evaluation of the ten-year quality agenda.* The Nuffield Trust, London.

Leatherman S and Sutherland K (2005) *The Quest for Quality in the NHS: a chartbook on quality of care in the UK.* Radcliffe Publishing, Oxford.

ONS (2004) Paper 1: Public Service Productivity. www.statistics.gov.uk

Panorama (2005) *What has Labour done for the NHS?* BBC, London.

Wanless D (2004) *Securing Good Health for the Whole Population Final Report.* HM Treasury, London.

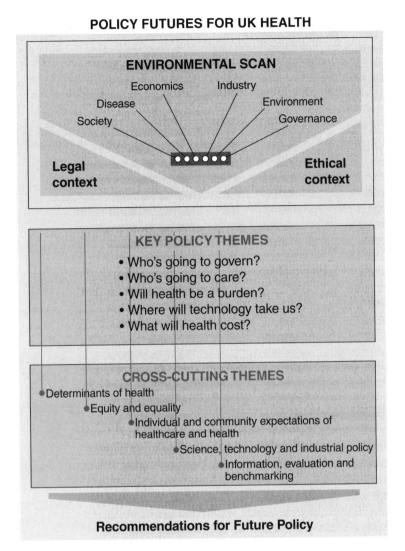

POLICY FUTURES FOR UK HEALTH

ENVIRONMENTAL SCAN

Economics   Industry

Disease   Environment

Society   Governance

**Legal
context**   **Ethical
context**

KEY POLICY THEMES

- Who's going to govern?
- Who's going to care?
- Will health be a burden?
- Where will technology take us?
- What will health cost?

CROSS-CUTTING THEMES

- Determinants of health
- Equity and equality
- Individual and community expectations of
  healthcare and health
- Science, technology and industrial policy
- Information, evaluation and
  benchmarking

Recommendations for Future Policy

Figure 1   Structure of the work represented in the book.

Part 1

Context

Chapter 1

Environmental scan

Linda Rosenstrøm Chang, Pam Garside, Suzanne Wait and Zoë Slote Morris

Society

Although globalisation has led to increasing wealth and opportunities afforded by economic developments in service and knowledge-based industries, sectors such as manufacturing, in which work can be exported to lower cost countries, have declined.

The role of women is continuously evolving with increased participation in the labour market, and family values and *household structures* are also continuing to change. The number of two-parent households is declining, while the number of three-generation households is increasing. This number is predicted to treble over the next 20 years so that one in every 25 households will be an extended family (Skipton Building Society, 2004). More people over the age of 16 are living alone (from 26.3% in 1991 to 31% in 2002) and half of the people living alone are elderly pensioners (ONS, 2002).

Citizens are increasingly defined as consumers of both private and public services. Although devolution has strengthened social choice at the home country level, local democracy within England has declined in significance and is being replaced by forms of consumer engagement. Alongside these developments is some recognition of growing inequalities in income, health and living conditions, as well as poverty and social exclusion within British society over the past 20 years. There is an urgent need to address these issues (Goodman and Shephard, 2002).

There has been an increase in *income inequality* over the last 20 years between socio-economic groups in the UK and there is still an income gender gap (Goodman and Shephard, 2002). The poorest tenth of the population has experienced little improvement in real levels compared to 25 years ago (Goodman and Shephard, 2002; Shephard, 2003). Among those who remain poor, the average shortfall in measured income below the poverty line has increased since 1996–97 (Brewer *et al.*, 2003).

- Two million children live in workless households.
- Lone-parent families, and couple households where both parents are out of work (with two or more children), are particularly at risk.
- Nearly 6% of the population live in accommodation with no heating and 12.3% live in an overcrowded home.
- Over one million adults of working age were paid less than £4.40 per hour in 2002.
- Around 10% of young adults (aged 16 to 24) were unemployed in 2003, which is double the rate among older workers (New Policy Institute, 2003b).

The *ageing* of the population continues to have implications for the disease burden faced by health and social care services (Khaw, 1999). Average life expectancy at birth is 75.8 years for men and 80.5 years for women, while healthy life expectancy is 69.1 years for men and 72.1 for women (WHO, 2004). Since 2001, there are more people over 60 than under 16 (Census, 2001). The dependency ratio is increasing, which means that a diminishing workforce is supporting a growing dependent population.

In England and Wales it is estimated that out of a total of six million carers, mostly caring for elderly parents or relatives, 5.2 million people provide unpaid care. A carer can be defined as 'a family member, friend or neighbour who is providing substantial or regular care to someone who is frail or ill or mentally or physically disabled' (NHS Scotland, 2003). One million of these unpaid carers give more than 50 hours weekly of care (Carers UK, 2005b). Almost two million carers are over 60 years of age. Although this provides a saving to the state of £57 billion annually (Carers UK, 2005a), reliance on informal care structures may be precarious as the burden of care will grow with the ageing of the population (Davies, 2003). The pension crisis delays retirement age, which in turn may mean fewer informal carers. Within the UK, Wales has the highest proportion of carers (11.7%), followed by the North East of England (11%). London has the lowest proportion (8.5%) of carers in England and Wales (Census, 2001; 2003).

The health needs of *immigrants* are different from the health needs of indigenous populations. Satisfaction with the NHS is related to ethnicity (CHI, 2004) and so, as the UK becomes more multicultural, satisfaction with the NHS could decline (Appleby and Rosete, 2003).

The increased *recruitment* needs of the NHS and the ageing of its workforce are creating major recruitment challenges for professional and support staff. Measures to replenish and expand the workforce are becoming critical to safeguarding future service delivery (University Hospital Birmingham, 2003). The impact of international labour mobility is being felt within the NHS: in 2003 two-thirds of the 1500 new full registrants on the General Medical Council (GMC) register were from overseas (Buchan, 2005), and 40% of registrations with the UKCC were from overseas (Nursing and Midwifery Council, 2004). The import of foreign-trained clinical staff may have an impact on the way patients are treated because of the variability in training standards and inconsistencies in staffing. A stable number of UK clinical staff is being recruited by other healthcare systems abroad, which means a steady loss of trained personnel (Lambert and Goldacre, 2002).

Defining 'poor' as living in a household where total income – adjusted for family size, children's age and housing costs – falls at or below 60% of the median income for all households in the UK, *childhood poverty* has fallen from 4.4 million by half a million since 1996–97 (Brewer *et al.*, 2003). A third of children in Wales and Scotland live in a low-income household, however, and childhood poverty is still on the rise in Scotland.

Babies born to parents from lower socio-economic groups or living in single-parent homes in the UK continue to be more likely to have low birthweight than those born to parents from higher socio-economic groups (New Policy Institute, 2003a). This has both a short-term and long-term impact on morbidity and life expectancy (Spenser, 1996). Teenage motherhood is ten times more likely in poorer neighbourhoods than in more affluent ones (Allison and Hall, 2001; DH, 2002). Other root causes of inequality associated with poorer health status are homelessness and exclusion from school.

The *voluntary sector* plays an important role in improving the health of the population. Its total income was £20 billion in 2004.

Evidence shows that *geographic location* is a predictor of poor health over and above personal and social characteristics such as employment history. Behavioural patterns and social circumstances are estimated to account for more than half of premature deaths in the US every year and similar patterns exist in Europe (IOM, 2003). There is also an observed relationship between social capital and health status. This is particularly important to people with mental health problems (Kawachi *et al.*, 1997; Lynch *et al.*, 2000; Phelan *et al.*, 2004). Crime is a greater problem in poorer areas and the consequences are more serious for more vulnerable members of society (Dodd *et al.*, 2004).

Several aspects of the *role of the patient* influence healthcare. Recognition of the individual's responsibility for healthy behaviour has been the foundation of the 'fully engaged' scenario, described in the Wanless report (2002). In the UK for example, although private gym membership is increasing (Hasler and Cooney, 2002), adults watch 3.7 hours of TV per day (BBC, 2004). In Scotland, people watch more television than any other region (Scottish Social Statistics, 2001). The amount of time children spend in front of the TV is increasing and this has been linked to the increasing levels of childhood obesity (Matheson *et al.*, 2004).

Health literacy has been defined as 'the degree in which individuals have the capacity to obtain, process, and understand the basic health information and services needed to make appropriate health decisions' (IOM, 2003). It is a critical determinant of health outcomes and several seminal reports have recognised the need to improve the 'health literacy' of patients and citizens (Detmer *et al.*, 2003). People engaging in risk behaviours may, however, be aware that what they are doing is unhealthy, but continue their behaviour to avoid deprivation. In some cases, they expect treatment and care in overcoming the unhealthy lifestyle.

There is growing recognition of the vital role that patients can play in self-care and self-education. In the case of 'expert patients' suffering from chronic diseases, they may be the ones best placed to set out their optimal course of care (DH, 2003). Increasing reliance by patients on the Internet as a source of information will have significant implications for how they approach their condition. There has been a rise in the use of NHS Direct, which expected 18 million calls in 2003/04 and NHS Direct Online, which received 4.6 million hits per month in 2001 (NHS Direct, 2001). Growing consumerism and individualism in society permeate into the health arena, modifying patients' expectations of care and shifting the balance of power in their relationship with healthcare providers (Coulter, 2002).

While patients may be expected to play a greater role in charting the course of their care, citizens and the public may also be expected to be further involved, or concerned, by the quality of services rendered by the NHS. The NHS is making more effort to try to understand patients' perspectives (CHI, 2004). In line with the 'fully engaged' scenario, the aim is to give patients greater choice in determining their own health, treatment and decisions about the NHS. Consumers only want choice if the provider is not acceptable in standard (Policy Commission on Public Services, 2004). There is more focus on devolving power to the locality.

In Census 2001, 18.2% of people in England and Wales reported that they suffered from a long-term illness or disability that limited their daily activities or the work they could do. Of these, 4.3 million were of working age, representing more than one-eighth of that age group. Only 13.3% of the population reported poor health in 1991 (Census, 2001; 2004).

Trends

As discussed above, some society-related trends include:

- increasing recognition of the economic and social determinants of health by the research community
- an ageing population, along with an increasing dependency ratio
- continuing unrecognised health needs of immigrant and ethnic minority households
- increasing health disparities in the last 20 years between the best- and worst-off in society
- a rise in individualism and consumerism in society and decline in local democracy
- changing household structures.

Current policy

It is a demographic fact that the population is ageing but the policy significance of what this will mean for society and the healthcare system is contested (Barnett Waddingham, 2002; Institute for Fiscal Studies, 2005; Prime Minister's Strategy Unit, 2005).

There is a continuing debate about reducing inequality in health, and individual versus state responsibility for health, with no clear outcome. Inequalities persist and have been linked with regional disparities: the line from the Severn to the Wash is said to indicate the levels of health and wellbeing. The current focus of government policy on reducing health inequalities was spearheaded by the publication of the *Report of the Independent Inquiry into Inequalities in Health* (Acheson, 1998). This report showed that poverty leads to poor health and in response the government launched a 20-year programme to eradicate child poverty (White, 1999). It also carried out a series of public consultations on reducing health inequalities (HM Treasury and DH, 2002) and budget spending reviews (HM Treasury, 2001; 2004b). Specific targets on reducing inequalities in the area of infant mortality were included in the Public Service Agreement between the DH and the Treasury (HM Treasury, 2004a). There has been much debate and controversy about the evidence base and the wisdom of these policies (Macintyre *et al.*, 2001; Oliver and Exworthy, 2003).

Recognising the links between life chances, deprivation and poor health, many policy actions have been implemented across different sectors, targeting specific vulnerable groups. These include the Welfare-to-Work programme for 18–25s, pension reform and the minimum income guarantee, child support reform and working family tax credits.

The Social Exclusion Unit was established by the Prime Minister to deal with some root causes of inequalities in England associated with poorer health status and there appears to be an increasing need for its activities.

Another focus of current policy is aimed at increasing public involvement in health (CHI, 2004; Opinion Leader Research, 2004). The Commission for Patient and Public Involvement in Health (CPPIH) was set up in January 2003 to promote public and patient involvement. One of the responsibilities of the CPPIH is to appoint members to the Patient and Public Involvement Forums, which have been created at local level within each PCT and NHS Trust in England. It was recently announced that the Commission will be abolished in 2006. Clarification as to how or whether it will be replaced is still not available.

Evidence of the connection between geography and health inequality has led to increasing policy action on tackling the social determinants of health (Marmot and Wilkinson, 1999; The Local Government Association *et al.,* 2004; UK Public Health Association, 2004). This increased awareness is apparent in the current focus on public health and the reduction of health risks, both in UK health policy and in international health policy forums (DH, 2004; Wanless, 2003; 2004; WHO, 2003). The impact of inequality of health is recognised, but the causes of poverty are not.

References

Acheson D (1998) *Report of the Independent Inquiry into Inequalities in Health.* The Stationery Office, London.

Allison R and Hall S (2001) Battle to cut teenage pregnancy rate. *The Guardian.* 22.2.01.

Appleby J and Rosete AA (2003) The NHS: keeping up with the public expectations? In: A Parke, J Curtice, K Thomson, L Jarvis and C Bromley (eds) *British Social Attitudes: the 20th Report – continuity and change over two decades.* Sage, London.

Barnett Waddingham (2002) The ageing population: burden or benefit? www.barnett-waddingham.co.uk

BBC (2004) Pay-TV outstripping advertising. news.bbc.co.uk

Brewer M, Clark T and Goodman A (2003) What really happened to child poverty in the UK under Labour's first term? *The Economic Journal.* **113**: 240–57.

Buchan J (2005) International recruitment of health professionals. *British Medical Journal.* **330**: 210.

Carers UK (2005a) Prime Minister defends record on carers. www.carersuk.org

Carers UK (2005b) Ten facts about caring. www.carersuk.org

Census 2001 (2001) Population report: demographics. www.statistics.gov.uk

Census 2001 (2003) Carers: 5.2 million carers in England and Wales. www.statistics.gov.uk

Census 2001 (2004) Census 2001: health, disability and provision of care. www.statistics.gov.uk

CHI (2004) *Unpacking the Patient's Perspective: variations in NHS patient experience in England.* Commission for Health Improvement, London.

Coulter A (2002) *The Autonomous Patient: ending paternalism in medical care.* The Nuffield Trust, London.

Davies C (2003) Introduction: a new workforce in the making? In: C Davies (ed.) *The Future Health Workforce.* Palgrave Macmillan, Basingstoke.

Detmer DE, Singleton PD, MacLeod A, Wait S, Taylor M and Ridgwell J (2003) *The Informed Patient: study report.* Cambridge University Health, Cambridge.

DH (2002) Government response to the first annual report of the Independent Advisory Group on teenage pregnancy. www.dh.gov.uk

DH (2003) The expert patient: a new approach to chronic disease management for the 21st century. www.dh.gov.uk

DH (2004) *Choosing Health: making healthier choices easier. Cmnd 6374.* Department of Health, London.

Dodd T, Nicholas S, Povey D and Walker A (2004) Home Office statistical bulletin: crime in England and Wales 2003/2004. www.homeoffice.gov.uk

Goodman A and Shephard A (2002) *Inequality and Living Standards in Britain: some facts.* Institute for Fiscal Studies, London.

Hasler P and Cooney A (2002) *Understanding the Health and Fitness Market.* MORI, London.

HM Treasury (2001) *Tackling Child Poverty: giving every child the best possible start in life – a pre-budget report document.* HM Treasury, London.

HM Treasury (2004a) *2004 Spending Review PSAs.* HM Treasury, London.

HM Treasury (2004b) *Spending Review: child poverty review.* HM Treasury, London.

HM Treasury and DH (2002) *Tackling Health Inequalities: summary of the 2002 cross-cutting review.* HM Treasury; DH, London.

Institute for Fiscal Studies (2005) Centre for Economic Research on Ageing: publications. www.ifs.org.uk/cera

IOM (2003) *Informing the Future: critical issues in health.* Institute of Medicine, London.

Kawachi I, Kennedy B and Lochner K (1997) A long live community: social capital as public health. *The American Prospect.* **35**: 56–9.

Khaw K (1999) How many, how old, how soon? *British Medical Journal.* **319**: 1350–2.

Lambert TW and Goldacre MJ (2002) Career destinations and view in 1998 of the doctors who qualified in the United Kingdom in 1993. *Medical Education.* **36**: 193–8.

Lynch J, Due P, Muntaner C and Smith GD (2000) Social capital: is it a good investment strategy for public health? *Journal of Epidemiology and Community Health.* **54**: 404–8.

Macintyre S, Chalmers I, Horton R and Smith R (2001) Using evidence to inform policy: case study. *British Medical Journal.* **322**: 222–5.

Marmot MG and Wilkinson R (1999) *Social Determinants of Health.* Oxford University Press, Oxford.

Matheson DM, Killen JD, Wang Y, Varady A and Robinson TN (2004) Children's food consumption during television viewing. *American Journal of Clinical Nutrition.* **79**(6): 1088–94.

New Policy Institute (2003a) Low birthweight babies. www.poverty.org.uk

New Policy Institute (2003b) Monitoring poverty and social exclusion: key facts. www.poverty.org.uk

NHS Direct (2001) *NHS Direct: a new gateway to healthcare.*

NHS Scotland (2003) Our definition of a carer. www.show.scot.nhs.uk

Nursing and Midwifery Council (2004) Statistical analysis of the register 1 April 2003 to 31 March 2004 (December 2004). www.nmc-uk.org

Oliver A and Exworthy M (2003) *Health Inequalities: evidence, policy and implementation – proceedings from a meeting of the Health Equity Network.* The Nuffield Trust, London.

ONS (2002) Living in Britain: results from the 2002 General Household Survey. Datasets 3.1 trends in household size: 1971 to 2002. www.statistics.gov.uk

Opinion Leader Research (2004) *Public Attitudes to Public Health Policy.* King's Fund; Health Development Agency; Department of Health, London.

Phelan JC, Link BG, Diez-Roux A, Kawachi I and Levin B (2004) 'Fundamental Causes' of Social Inequalities in Mortality: a test of the theory. *Journal of Health and Social Behavior.* **45**(3): 265–85.

Policy Commission on Public Services (2004) *Making Public Services Personal: a new contract for public services – The independent Policy Commission on Public Services report to the National Consumer Council.* Policy Commission on Public Services, London.

Prime Minister's Strategy Unit (2005) *Strategic Audit: progress and challenges for the UK.* Prime Minister's Strategy Unit, London.

Scottish Social Statistics (2001) 2001 Scottish social statistics. www.scotland.gov.uk

Shephard A (2003) *Inequality under the Labour government.* Institute for Fiscal Studies, London.

Skipton Building Society (2004) *Financing Your Future.* Skipton Building Society, Skipton.

Spencer N (1996) *Poverty and Child Health.* Radcliffe Medical Press, Oxford.

The Local Government Association, The UK Public Health Association and The NHS Confederation (2004) *Realising the Potential for the Public's Health.* The Local Government Association, London.

UK Public Health Association (2004) *State of Britain's Health: poverty and inequality.* UK Public Health Association, London.

University Hospital Birmingham (2003) *Corporate Strategy 2003–2010.* University Hospital Birmingham, Birmingham.

Wanless D (2002) *Securing our Future Health: taking a long-term view.* HM Treasury, London.

Wanless D (2003) *Securing Good Health for the Whole Population: population health trends.* HM Treasury, London.

Wanless D (2004) *Securing Good Health for the Whole Population: final report.* HM Treasury, London.

White M (1999) PM's 20-year target to end poverty. *The Guardian.* 19.3.99.

WHO (2003) *The World Health Report 2003: shaping the future.* World Health Organization, Geneva.

WHO (2004) Countries. www.who.int

Disease

The overall burden of disease has continued to shift from the young to the old, and from communicable to non-communicable chronic disease, since 2000 (Yach *et al.*, 2004). Chronic disease – including cardiovascular disease, stroke, cancer, diabetes, respiratory disease, HIV/AIDS, tuberculosis, neuropsychiatric disorders, musculo-skeletal disease and osteoporosis – represents the main burden of mortality and morbidity within the UK (Wagner and Groves, 2002).

In a cross-national UK survey of self-reported *general health*, 74% of adults found themselves to be in good health (Census, 2001; 2003). Life expectancy at age 65 is 15.6 years in males and 18.9 years in females (OECD, 2003). In the UK, infant mortality rates and rates of low-birthweight children are higher than in other OECD countries (2003). Although comparable with other OECD countries (2003), there are relatively poor health outcomes in coronary heart disease (CHD), cancer and respiratory disease (Wanless, 2003). Coronary heart disease and strokes account for a third of all deaths in men and a fifth of all deaths in women aged 65 years and under, although mortality rates from CHD have been declining over the last three years due to statins. Deaths from respiratory disease are increasing (British Thoracic Society, 2000). Trends in cancer predict a steady rise in incidence, however mortality rates from cancer have been decreasing for the past few years due to improved treatment (NHS, 2003).

Smoking has remained at the same level since the 1990s and has been identified as the single greatest cause of avoidable ill health and untimely death in the UK (ASH, 2005; Department of Health Social Services and Public Safety 2000; Murray 2005). The uptake of smoking among the young continues and 10% of 11–16 year olds smoke regularly. Despite this, it is predicted that only 8% of the UK population will be smokers by 2050 (Future Foundation, 2005). In 1980, *alcohol* accounted for 2% of deaths among 15–44 year olds compared with 7% of deaths among men and 6% among women today. In the last decade, among young men, there has almost been a doubling of alcohol-related deaths (Prime Minister's Strategy Unit, 2004). *Drug abuse* shows little variation in usage between 1994 and 2000, although there has been an increase in cocaine usage (Jeffery *et al.*, 2002). Drug use is practised across all socio-economic groups, but the majority of drug abusers is found among the lower socio-economic groups (Jupp *et al.*, 1997).

The UK has the highest rate of overweight and *obese* people in the EU, which will be an important determinant of future disease patterns (House of Commons Health Committee, 2004; Royal College of Physicians *et al.*, 2004). The proportion of obese adults rose from 13 to 21% for men and 15 to 24% for women between 1991/92 and 2001. The proportion of obese children rose from 12.1% in 1996 to 15.6% in 2001. If current trends continue, conservative estimates are that at least one-third of adults, one-fifth of boys, and one-third of girls will be obese by 2020 (NAO, 2001). Obesity is thought to reduce life expectancy by, on average, nine years and accounted for 30 000 deaths in 1998 (NAO, 2001). Indeed, after more than a century of rapidly rising life expectancy, today's young people will have shorter lives than their parents (BBC, 2004; BMA, 2003; The Fabian Society, 2003). Coronary heart disease, stroke, joint problems and the most common form of diabetes (type 2) are direct consequences of obesity. More than 3% of the English population suffers from diabetes and this number is rising (Gale, 2003; Wanless, 2004).

Accidents, including head injuries, are the biggest threat to life for children and young people. They are also a major cause of death and disability in older people. Overall, accidental deaths have been reduced by 20% between 1980 and 2000 (ONS, 2005). The main cause of death for children under 15, accounting for 50% of all injury deaths, is traffic accidents (Monaghan *et al.*, 2002). There has been a minor increase in traffic accidents, with Northern Ireland having the worst record in the UK and rates in Scotland rising slightly (BBC, 2002b).

Despite the main burden of disease falling on chronic disease, some *infectious diseases* are on the rise. Tuberculosis (TB) has increased by 25% over the last ten years, though people are at higher risk if they have lived in parts of the world where it is more common. In England, two-thirds of TB patients were born outside the UK (DH, 2004e). Human immunodeficiency virus (HIV) infection is also rising, although AIDS occurrence and death from AIDS remain stable (National Statistics, 2003). There is a general rise in sexually transmitted diseases, of which chlamydia is the commonest and fastest spreading in the UK: one in ten sexually active young women has chlamydia, which can cause infertility if untreated. The increase in multi-drug resistance is also modifying the character and occurrence of many infectious diseases and posing huge challenges to antibiotic therapies against common pathogens (HPA, 2004c). The UK has the highest rates of bacterial isolates of *staphylococcus aureus* resistance in Europe (43.9% in 2002) and 9% of patients in NHS hospitals suffer from an infection acquired while on wards or in surgery (NAO, 2004). There is an increase in the incidence of hepatitis B and C in the UK, especially for drug users (BBC, 2003; United Kingdom Parliament, 2001). In England and Wales, hepatitis B has doubled over the last decade (HPA, 2004a) while hepatitis C has risen 26 times between 1992 and 2003 (HPA, 2004b). Each year, it is estimated that as many as 5.5 million people in the UK may suffer from food-borne illnesses (Foodlink, 2004). Food poisoning peaked in 1997 but is now declining, largely due to animal vaccination programmes which have reduced the number of red meat and salmonella infections (BBC, 2002a).

At any given time, one in six adults suffers from a common *mental health* problem, such as depression or anxiety (Mental Health Foundation, 2004; Psychiatric Morbidity Survey and Office of Population, 2000). Poor mental health is increasing in children and young people (BMA, 2003). Depression is one of the more common reasons for visits to the doctor, and is on the rise. The total cost of mental health problems has been estimated at £32 billion, of which £12 billion is attributed to lost employment and productivity (Mental Health Foundation, 2004). Suicide rates are falling in England, but not in Scotland, which now has a fifth of all young adult suicides in the UK. Suicide is the second most common cause of death in young men, claiming more lives than cancer (The Samaritans, 1997) and depression is linked to at least 3000 out of the 4000 annual suicides in England.

Neuropsychiatric disorders were found to account for over one-fifth of total disability-adjusted life years (DALYs) in Europe, a composite indicator of disease burden (WHO, 2001). Dementia may eventually strike 85% of the population (Foresight, 2000). The trend is towards the increasing medicalisation of conditions such as attention deficit disorder (ADD) in children, hyperactivity and milder age-related cognitive impairments (Foresight, 2000).

Zoonotic diseases (diseases that pass from animals to humans, such as BSE and bird flu) are emerging (IOM, 2003). They are difficult to manage and public health governance is becoming more important as diseases cross geographical borders.

Worldwide public health surveillance has become an essential means of under-standing and controlling disease incidence and transmission patterns for HIV/AIDS, SARS and bio-terrorism (HPA, 2005).

The rising threat of *bio-terrorism* since the events of 11 September 2001 has led to the establishment of a European Task Force on Bio-Terrorism. The European Commission has been working with WHO and G8 to ensure global preparedness for possible threats (IOM, 2003).

Health inequalities have been worsening over the last 20 years (Drever *et al.*, 2004; Drever *et al.*, 1996). Social, economic, geographical, regional and ethnic variations in inequalities are apparent in life expectancy and in the incidence and outcomes of cancer, mental health, accidents, obesity, diabetes, heart disease, strokes and TB. The poorest people in society are hardest hit by major causes of death; they are ill more often and they die sooner. Mortality rates are 70% higher in the most deprived areas than the most affluent. It has been estimated that a concerted effort to improve the state of health of the poorest people to bring it up to the level of the most affluent could reduce hospital admissions by 6%, saving the NHS up to £850 million annually (HM Treasury, 2002; Wanless, 2003).

Trends

As discussed above, some health-related trends include:

- improvements regarding smoking and road safety, and better treatment of HIV/AIDS, cancer and cardiovascular diseases
- non-communicable, chronic disease now the main burden of disease
- an increase in alcohol and drug misuse, obesity and diabetes
- a significant increase in anti-microbial drug resistance
- an increasing burden of mental illness
- infectious diseases (re)-emerging, often through foodborne routes
- the emergence of zoonotic diseases globally
- increasing social, geographical, economic and ethnic inequalities in health.

Current policy

The rise in chronic illnesses has severe implications for the organisation and delivery of care. It has contributed to policy plans to build greater collaboration between social and healthcare services. Standardising practice through national guidelines and recommendations has also been the focus of recent policy. Since 1998, a rolling programme of National Service Frameworks (NSFs) has been and is being estab-lished in England and Wales. The NSFs set out guidelines for treatment protocols and organisation of care for given conditions. It is hoped that these will raise standards of care across the NHS, tackling morbidity and mortality in priority areas.

The government has developed dedicated strategies to tackle the major causes of morbidity and mortality, namely in the areas of heart disease and strokes, accidents, cancer and mental health. *The NHS Cancer Plan: three year progress report – maintaining the momentum* (2003) sets targets to reduce the mortality rate from cancer in people under 75 years by 20% by 2010 against a 1995–97 baseline. It also addresses inequality and makes commitments to improve access to services throughout the country (NAO, 2005).

In 2001, the Treasury commissioned an independent Long-Term Health Trends Review, led by Derek Wanless. In *Securing Our Future Health: taking a long-term view* (Wanless, 2002), the report made use of scenario planning to illustrate how resources could be used in the future in the UK and clarified the long-term resource requirements needed. The report described three scenarios: 'solid progress', 'slow uptake' and 'fully engaged'. In the preferred, fully engaged scenario, the public is most engaged, health improves dramatically, life expectancy increases and people trust the health service, although it is questionable whether the fully engaged person will come into being (Health Foundation, 2003; Shepherd, 2004; Walker, 2002; Watt, 2004). Following the report, the government committed greater funding for NHS up to 2008 (Guardian, 2002).

The NHS Improvement Plan: putting people at the heart of public services (DH, 2004d) set out government plans for further modernisation of, and priorities for, the NHS to 2008. It promises more 'personalised care' and a greater focus on wellbeing. *National Standards, Local Action: health and social care standards and planning framework 2005/06 to 2007/08* (DH, 2004c) also includes priorities for tackling disease, inequalities and services, and long-term conditions receive increased priority.

The final Wanless report, *Securing Good Health for the Whole Population* (Wanless, 2004), states that the English NHS must be transformed from a 'sickness service' into a 'health service', with more emphasis on public health and 'improving the health of the [whole] population, not just treating the diseases of individual patients'.

Although there has been an increased focus on lifestyle changes in relation to health in the last few years, more could be achieved. The *Alcohol Harm Reduction Strategy for England* (Prime Minister's Strategy Unit, 2004) proposes that industry should be more responsible, but no targets have been defined and no supporting legislation is planned. Similarly, strategies for obesity, such as *Reducing and Preventing Obesity: everything must change* make the assumption that the DH cannot 'be expected to "cure" the problem' alone and emphasises lifestyle changes to reduce obesity (House of Commons Health Committee, 2004). The *Choosing Health: making healthier choices easier* White Paper (DH, 2004a) refers to individual more than governmental responsibility for health, and to governmental responsibility in relation to multinational corporations and their (food and drinks) products. The White Paper does recognise work being undertaken in other arenas, mentioning the SureStart and New Deal programmes for improving health and reducing inequalities. These programmes provide some evidence of cross-departmental work.

The existing Mental Health Act dates from 1983. The new Mental Health Draft Bill of September 2004 is controversial, setting, among other things, criteria for when patients can be detained (DH, 2004b). A parliamentary committee reported in March 2005 that the Scottish Mental Health Act serves as a good example, that the definition of mental health should be broad but with exclusions to prevent inappropriate use, and that the individual has the ability to decide about whether he needs treatment (Joint Committee on the Draft Mental Health Bill, 2005). New legislation has been enacted in Scotland (Rushmer and Hallam, 2004). The *National Suicide Prevention Strategy for England* (DH, 2002) is part of the government's plan to reduce the suicide rate by at least 20% by 2010. Housing and unemployment are mentioned as risk factors leading to poor mental health, but it is not entirely clear how the government intends to tackle these issues.

There is a greater awareness of unknown threats and the need to manage them. An Emergency Planning Coordination Unit (EPCU) within the DH is responsible for the coordination of contingency planning to maintain the state of readiness of the NHS to respond to major incidents. The Global Health Security Initiative aims to mobilise resources in a global health security drive to deal with any deliberate release of communicable disease agents or chemical substances. The European Centre for Disease Prevention and Control (ECDC) was created following the SARS epidemic (European Commission, 2003; Wellcome Trust, 2004).

References

ASH (2005) Basic facts two: smoking and disease. www.ash.org.uk

BBC (2002a) Rise in severe food poisoning. http://news.bbc.co.uk

BBC (2002b) Road deaths rise slightly. http://news.bbc.co.uk

BBC (2003) Call for hepatitis B vaccination. http://news.bbc.co.uk

BBC (2004) US questions global obesity plan. http://news.bbc.co.uk

BMA (2003) *Adolescent Health*. British Medical Association Board of Science and Education, BMA, London.

British Thoracic Society (2000) *The Burden of Lung Disease: a statistics report from the British Thoracic Society*. British Thoracic Society, London.

Census 2001 (2003) Carers: 5.2 million carers in England and Wales. www.statistics.gov.uk

Department of Health Social Services and Public Safety (2000) *Investing for Health: a consultation paper*. Ministerial Group on Public Health, Belfast.

DH (2002) *National Suicide Prevention Strategy for England*. Department of Health, London.

DH (2004a) *Choosing Health: making healthier choices easier. Cmnd 6374*. The Stationery Office, London.

DH (2004b) *Draft Mental Health Bill. Cmnd 6305–1*. The Stationery Office, London.

DH (2004c) *National Standards, Local Action: health and social care standards and planning framework 2005/06 to 2007/08*. Department of Health, London.

DH (2004d) *NHS Improvement Plan: putting people at the heart of public services*. Department of Health, London.

DH (2004e) *Stopping Tuberculosis in England: an action plan from the Chief Medical Officer*. Department of Health, London.

Drever F, Doran T and Whitehead M (2004) Exploring the relation between class, gender, and self-rated general health using the new socioeconomic classification: a study using data from the 2001 census. *Journal of Epidemiology and Community Health*. **58**: 7.

Drever F, Whitehead M and Roden M (1996) Current patterns and trends in male mortality by social class (based on occupation). *Population Trends*. **86**: 4.

European Commission (2003) *European Centre for Disease Prevention and Control*. http://europa.eu.int

Foodlink (2004) Food poisoning. www.foodlink.org.uk

Foresight (2000) *Healthcare*. Foresight, London.

Future Foundation (2005) *Up in Smoke: quitting smoking in the 21st century*. Future Foundation, London.

Gale E (2003) Is there really an epidemic of type 2 diabetes? *The Lancet*. **362**: 9383.

Health Foundation (2003) The Health Foundation: submission to the Wanless Review on population health. www.health.org.uk

HM Treasury (2002) *2002 Spending Review: new public spending plans 2003–2006*. HM Treasury, London.

House of Commons Health Committee (2004) *Obesity. Third Report of Session 2003–04*. TSO, London.

HPA (2004a) Hepatitis B notifications: England and Wales, by region, 1990–2003. www.hpa.org.uk

HPA (2004b) Hepatitis C laboratory report: England and Wales, by region, 1992–2003. www.hpa.org.uk

HPA (2004c) *Staphylococcus aureus*. www.hpa.org.uk

HPA (2005) Surveillance, response and coordination. www.hpa.org.uk

IOM (2003) *Informing the Future: critical issues in health*. Institute of Medicine, London.

Jeffery D, Klein A and King L (2002) *United Kingdom: drug situation 2001*. European Monitoring Centre for Drugs and Drug Addiction, Lisbon.

Joint Committee on the Draft Mental Health Bill (2005) *Joint Committee on the Draft Mental Health Bill – First Report*. The United Kingdom Parliament, London.

Jupp B, Perry H and Lasky K (1997) *The Substance of Youth: the role of drugs in young peoples' lives today*. Joseph Rowntree Foundation, York.

Mental Health Foundation (2004) Statistics on mental health. www.mentalhealth.org.uk

Monaghan S, Huws D and Na M (2002) *The Case for a new UK Health of the People Act*. The Nuffield Trust, London.

Murray E (2005) *Current Motions: no smoking day 2005*. Scottish Parliament, Edinburgh.

NAO (2001) Tackling obesity in England. www.nao.org.uk

NAO (2004) *Improving Patient Care by Reducing the Risk of Hospital Acquired Infection: a progress report*. National Audit Office, London.

NAO (2005) *The NHS Cancer Plan: a progress report*. National Audit Office, London.

NHS (2003) *The NHS Cancer Plan: three year progress report – maintaining the momentum*. Department of Health, London.

OECD (2003) *Health At A Glance: OECD indicators 2003*. OECD, Paris.

ONS (2003) *HIV and AIDS*. www.statistics.gov.uk

ONS (2005) *Deaths from Injury and Poisoning: external cause and year of registration or occurrence, 1901–2000*. www.statistics.gov.uk

Prime Minister's Strategy Unit (2004) *Alcohol Harm Reduction Strategy For England*. Cabinet Office, London.

Psychiatric Morbidity Survey and Office of Population (2000) Lifetime experience of stressful life events by type of event and gender, 2000: Social Trends 32. www.statistics.gov.uk

Royal College of Physicians, Faculty of Public Health and Royal College of Paediatrics and Child Health (2004) *Storing Up Problems: the medical case for a slimmer nation*. Royal College of Physicians, London.

Royal College of Physicians, Royal College of Paediatrics and Child Health and Faculty of Public Health (2004) *Reducing and Preventing Obesity – everything must change*. Royal College of Physicians, London.

Rushmer M and Hallam A (2004) *Mental Health Law Research Programme: analysis of responses to consultation*. Scottish Executive Social Research, Edinburgh.

Shepherd J (2004) *'There is more to life than health'– a response to the Wanless article*. Academy of Medical Sciences, London.

The Fabian Society (2003) *All's Well that Starts Well*. The Fabian Society, London.

The Guardian (2002) NHS finance 2002–03: the issue explained. http://society. guardian.co.uk

The Samaritans (1997) *Exploring the Taboo*. The Samaritans, Ewell, Surrey.

United Kingdom Parliament (2001) *MEMORANDUM 2. Submitted by Action on Hepatitis C. Current UK drug policy will increase drug-related deaths from bloodborne virus infections.* United Kingdom Parliament, London.

Wagner EH and Groves T (2002) Care for chronic diseases. *British Medical Journal.* **325**: 913–14.

Walker D (2002) The Wanless NHS has a moral heart. *The Guardian.* 17.4.02.

Wanless D (2002) *Securing our Future Health: taking a long-term view.* HM Treasury, London.

Wanless D (2003) *Securing Good Health for the Whole Population: population health trends.* HM Treasury, London.

Wanless D (2004) *Securing Good Health for the Whole Population: final report.* HM Treasury, London.

Watt G (2004) *Life-style: your health in your hands – a response to the Wanless article.* The Academy of Medical Sciences, London.

Wellcome Trust (2004) *Public Health Sciences: challenges and opportunities. Report of the Public Health Sciences Working Group convened by the Wellcome Trust.* The Wellcome Trust, London.

WHO (2001) *Mental Health: new understanding, new hope.* World Health Organization, Geneva.

Yach D, Hawkes C, Gold C and Hofman K (2004) The global burden of chronic diseases. *Journal of the American Medical Association.* **291**: 21.

Environment

The environment can be defined as 'people, their local environment and the collective influences of society on individual life chances' (Palmer *et al.*, 1999). It is not easy to isolate the particular effects of the natural, built and socio-economic environment but this section examines the first two factors to show how housing, transport and economic policies, particularly regarding redistribution of wealth, affect health.

Changes in weather, climate and rising sea levels, as a consequence of *global warming*, will affect the health and wellbeing of individuals and populations. In 2000, an estimated 150 000 deaths worldwide were attributable to factors such as heat, droughts and floods caused by climate change (McMichael *et al.*, 2003). Climate change may modify the spatial and temporal distribution of a range of infectious diseases – either directly or through changes in disease vectors or hosts (EEHC Secretariat, 2003) – while ozone depletion is associated with a continuing upward trend in skin cancers (Diffey, 2004).

The emission of greenhouse gases is declining steadily in accordance with EU agreements – such as the Gothenburg targets for total emission and the European Commission National Emission Ceilings Directive (NECD) for total emissions (ONS, 2004) – and emissions from industry are declining too. There are more air pollutants, however, due to more trips made particularly by air and car, and less trips made by foot or bicycle (Department for Transport, 2004). The indications for switching to diesel fuels are contradictory since these reduce greenhouse gasses but increase particulates and hence allergies.

Although people who are exposed to air pollution are more likely to die from heart disease than from respiratory disease (Pope *et al.*, 2004), studies have shown there may be a link between air pollution and other serious conditions, including lung cancer and strokes (Committee on the Medical Effects of Air Pollutants, 1998; BMJ, 2002). More recently, studies have shown a link between air pollution and life expectancy (WHO, 2004; European Commission, 2005a).

In May 2005, the European Commission introduced a new strategy to reduce the threat to health by air pollution. British scientists are carrying out a study to determine whether changing the way towns and cities are designed could improve residents' health. According to a Friends of the Earth study, poor areas have more pollution, with one out of every two municipal waste incinerators in England located in the poorest 10% of the country (BBC, 2004b). Eighty per cent of the UK population lives within two kilometres of a current or closed landfill site. There is a 1% increase in the risk of birth defects to babies born near a landfill site and this increases to 7% for those near a hazardous waste site (Elliott *et al.*, 2001).

The UK has the highest asthma rates in the EU by far: at 13.8% it is almost double the EU 7.2% average (Directorate General Health and Consumer Protection, 2003). In addition, one in three children and young adults in the UK suffers from allergies (BBC, 2004a). The most common form of asthma is the result of airways inflammation caused by exposure to an environmental allergen (McMorran *et al.*, 2005). Pollution, wall-to-wall carpets, poor housing and occupation are some of the factors that can cause asthma.

The increased use of renewable – especially wind, solar and photovoltaic – energy in the UK will have benefits for health (Sims, 2004). Health and environmental benefits easily make up for the higher costs associated with renewable energy use (EEHC Secretariat, 2003).

An increasing number of *chemicals* are entering the global market. There is increased surveillance of the connection between chemicals and health in the UK, and increased research being conducted to better understand the impact of this (HPA, 2004; WWF, 2004). An EU measure called REACH (Registration, Evaluation and Authorisation of Chemicals) has been proposed (European Commission, 2005b), which is intended to impose strict regulation on Europe's chemical industry. It will require new laboratory tests for 30 000 separate chemicals currently in production in Europe.

There is little definitive data linking human reproductive disorders or cancers with exposure to environmental synthetic chemicals and understanding of their potential to cause harm is incomplete. The reproductive effects of environmental chemicals in (aquatic) wildlife, however, are well established and may provide pointers for human effects (Sharpe and Irvine, 2004).

According to WHO, for many years the *housing* environment has been acknowledged as one of the main settings that affects human health. Problems include poor indoor air quality, accidents, high noise levels, high humidity, low temperature, asbestos, volatile organic components and overcrowding. Anxiety, depression and lower life expectancy increase in correlation to the number of housing problems experienced (Wilkinson, 1999; Olsen, 2003; Healthcare Commission, 2004). Despite significant literature suggesting a link between poor housing and health, the evidence is weak. Housing interventions and improvements do not always show parallel improvements in health (Wilkinson, 1999; Bonnefoy *et al.,* 2003). Furthermore, when they have been shown to have a positive affect on health, there have been limits to the generalisation of the findings (Thomson, 2001; Thomson *et al.,* 2003).

The DH has nevertheless established the link between disease and housing in the initiatives of *Housing, Health and Social Care for Older People* (DH, 2004). Work is being undertaken to study the relationship between environmental quality and deprivation, and multiple health effects. Urbanisation has particular risks for health, with deterioration of community for those located at the edges of urban sprawl due to loss of access to facilities. Urban growth is also associated with increased alcoholism, drug use and violence (Asthana *et al.,* 2002).

Trends

As discussed above, some health-related trends in the environment include:

- climate change caused by global warming
- a continuing upward trend in skin cancers due to ozone depletion and increasing time spent outdoors
- a rise in the number of allergies in the UK
- increasing numbers of chemicals entering the global market
- some improvements in air quality due to reductions in the major sources of pollution.

Current policy

Many environmental policies depend on global agreement making environmental issues, and their impact on health, foreign policy issues. While there is a generally low level of enthusiasm in the UK for EU environmental controls, action at this level is crucial for future global accord. The EU Maastricht Agreement noted the need to subject all public policy to health impact assessment, although the impact is contested (Greer, 2005). Issues should be managed nationally and internationally (regarding emissions, for example) rather than locally.

Another concern is that policies are not sufficiently improving the environmental situation. A recent report by the Sustainable Development Commission stated that the UK is unlikely to meet its target for carbon emissions by 2010: the government's efforts have proved 'disappointing' on climate change; waste management in the UK was 'dreadful' (the commission's harshest remark in the five-year review) with recycling rates among the lowest in Europe; and traffic congestion was also 'dreadful', with Britons spending more time commuting than any of their European counterparts. The authors of the report complained that ministers did not make a connection between public health and sustainable development when drawing up policy (Sustainable Development Commission, 2003).

Securing the Future, a revised strategy for the UK on sustainable development, came out of the consultation *Taking it On* (DEFRA, 2004; HM Government, 2005). The four priority areas for the UK are sustainable consumption and production, climate change and energy, natural resource protection and environmental enhancement, and sustainable communities. The emphasis is on changing behaviour in all of these areas.

The Water Act was passed in 2003 (the UK is one of the most water-stressed countries in the world), as was the Household Waste and Recycling Act and the Sustainable Energy Act. Considering the provisions of the Environment Protection Act (1995) and the lack of cross-departmental co-operation, there appears to be no clear leadership at all levels dealing with the health impact and the environment. This may change when the UK has the EU presidency later in 2005 (Green Alliance, 2004). Two bills, which would have an effect on renewable energy, are currently before Parliament: Renewable Energy and Renewable Heat.

The European Commission published an *Environment and Health Strategy* with the overall aim to reduce diseases caused by environmental factors in Europe. In its first phase from 2003–10, the focus will be on four key health concerns: childhood respiratory diseases, neurodevelopment disorders, childhood cancers and endocrine disruptor effects.

The Transport and Health Study Group studies the links between transport and health. It examines the promotion of walking and cycling, the promotion of less polluting alternatives to motor vehicles, transport for disabled people, transport for health purposes, the impact of transport on local communities, road safety, the impact of transport availability on social exclusion and the role of transport in promoting healthy lifestyles, for example in accessing the countryside or sources of healthy food (Stockport NHS, 2004).

References

Asthana S, Curtis S, Duncan C and Gould M (2002) Themes in British health geography at the end of the century: a review of published research 1998–2000. *Social Science & Medicine.* **55**: 167–73.

BBC (2004a) Allergy surge to be investigated. http://news.bbc.co.uk/1/hi/health/3475279.stm. Accessed: 23 March 2004.

BBC (2004b) Poor areas 'have more pollution'. http://news.bbc.co.uk/1/hi/health/3394793.stm. Accessed: 25 March 2004.

BMJ (2002) Air pollution and short-term mortality. Editorial. *British Medical Journal.* **324**: 691–2.

Bonnefoy XR, Braubach M, Moissonnier, B, Monolbaev K and Röbbel N (2003) *Housing and Health in Europe: preliminary results of a pan-European study.* World Health Organization's Regional Office for Europe, Bonn.

Committee on the Medical Effects of Air Pollutants (1998) *Quantification of the Effects of Air Pollution on Health in the United Kingdom.* Department of Health, London.

DEFRA (2004) *Taking it On. Developing UK sustainable development strategy together. A consultation paper.* Department for Environment, Food and Rural Affairs, London.

DH (2004) *Housing, Health and Social Care for Older People: building the links.* Department of Health, London.

Department for Transport (2004) Driving Force: four fifths of distance travelled is by car. http://www.statistics.gov.uk/cci/nugget.asp?id=24. Accessed: 31 March 2004.

Diffey B (2004) Climate change, ozone depletion and the impact of ultraviolet exposure on human skin. *Physical and Medical Biology.* **49**(1): 1–11.

Directorate General Health and Consumer Protection (2003) *Health, Food and Alcohol and Safety.* European Commission, Brussels.

Elliott P, Briggs D, Morris S, de Hoogh C, Hurt C, Jensen TK, Maitland I, Richardson S, Wakefield J and Jarup L (2001) Risk of adverse birth outcomes in populations living near landfill sites. *British Medical Journal.* **323**: 363–8.

European Commission (2005a) Air pollution: new EU limits are now in force: small airborne particles like diesel soot should be reduced. http://64.233.183.104/search?q=cache:NCfJcMpKVfAJ:europa.eu.int/luxembourg/docs/023-2005_en.doc+european+commission+air+pollution+life+expectancy&hl=en&start=2&client=safari. Accessed: 21 March 2005.

European Commission (2005b) REACH: Commission supports search for balanced solutions to advance progress on new chemicals policy. http://europa.eu.int/rapid/pressReleasesAction.do?reference=IP/05/60&format=HTML&aged=0&language=EN&guiLanguage=en. Accessed: 21 March 2005.

European Environment and Health Committee (EEHC) Secretariat (2003) *Energy, Sustainable Development and Health.* World Health Organization, Copenhagen.

Green Alliance (2004) *Setting the Agenda: environmental leadership for the UK presidency of the EU. Final report to DEFRA.* Green Alliance, IEEP, DEFRA, London.

Greer S (2005) *The New EU Health Policy and the NHS Systems.* The Nuffield Trust, London.

Healthcare Commission (2004) *State of Healthcare Report.* Healthcare Commission, London.

HM Government (2005) *Securing the Future – UK Government sustainable development strategy.* HM Government, London.

HPA (2004) Chemicals and poisons. http://www.natfocus.uwic.ac.uk/. Accessed: 25 March 2004.

McMichael AJ, Campbell-Lendrum DH, Corvalán CF and Ebi KL (2003) *Climate Change and Human Health – risks and responses.* World Health Organization, Geneva.

McMorran J, Crowther DC, McMorran S, Prince C, YoungMin S, Pleat J and Wacogne I (2005) Types of asthma. http://www.gpnotebook.co.uk/simplepage.cfm?ID=1925906359&linkID=3004&cook=yes. Accessed: 15 March 2005.

Olsen N (2003) *Engaging Health Professionals in Action on Unhealthy Housing.* Healthy Housing: promoting good health conference, 19–21 March 2003. University of Warwick, Warwick, p. 13.

ONS (2004) *The Environment in Your Pocket.* National Statistics Department for Environment Food and Rural Affairs, London.

Palmer S, Burr M, Coleman G, Jones P, Kay D, Matthews I, Thomas D, Salmon R and Watkins J (1999) *A Review of Trends in the Natural and Built Environment.* The Nuffield Trust, London.

Pope CA, Burnett RT, Thurston GD, Thun MJ, Calle EE, Krewski D and Godleski JJ (2004) Cardiovascular mortality and long-term exposure to particulate air pollution. Epidemiological evidence of general pathophysiological pathways of disease. *Circulation.* **109**: 71–7.

Sharpe RM and Irvine DS (2004) How strong is the evidence of a link between environmental chemicals and adverse effects on human reproductive health? *British Medical Journal.* **328**: 447–51.

Sims REH (2004) Renewable energy: a response to climate change. *Solar Energy.* **76**(1): 9–17.

Stockport NHS (2004) Transport and Health Study Group. http://www.stockport.nhs.uk/thsg/. Accessed: 19 May 2004.

Sustainable Development Commission (2003) *UK Climate Change Programme: a policy audit.* Sustainable Development Commission, London.

Thomson H (2001) Health effects of housing improvement: systematic review of intervention studies. *British Medical Journal.* **323**: 187–90.

Thomson H, Petticrew M and Douglas M (2003) Health impact assessment of housing improvements: incorporating research evidence. *Journal of Epidemiology and Community Health.* **57**(1): 11–16.

WHO (2004) One in three child deaths in Europe due to environment: new WHO study details devastating effects. http://www.euro.who.int/mediacentre/PR/2004/20040617_1. Accessed: 21 March 2005.

Wilkinson D (1999) *Poor Housing and Ill Health.* Central Research Unit, The Scottish Office, Edinburgh.

WWF (2004) Chemicals and health campaign. http://www.wwf.org.uk/chemicals/. Accessed: 25 March 2004.

Governance

Trends in governance that are relevant to UK health policy operate at global, EU, UK and health-system levels.

Globalisation is a powerful trend affecting the governance of health systems, as nation states need to address the impact of the internationalisation of health risk, increasing global interdependence and the uneven distribution of the costs and benefits of health policy. New and re-emerging diseases such as SARS and Avian Flu have met with globalised reactions and responses (WHO, 2004). There are many challenges associated with global labour markets, however, and overall the global governance of public health remains weak in relation to macro-economic and trade policies (Ham, 2004).

Within the *European Union,* although the Maastricht and Amsterdam Treaties introduced common guidance on public health and health information, governance over health and healthcare systems rests within the competency of each individual member state. This separation continues in the proposed EU Constitution and, if enacted, the new constitution will replace these previous treaties. EU policies and guidance are thus likely to be of increasing importance in the field of public health and will provide the base for common action on public health issues.

The EU has also invested significant efforts in strengthening its public health capabilities. It has plans for the creation of a European Centre for Disease Control in the near future and it initiated the Programme of Community Action in public health in 2003 (European Commission, 2002b). The programme, which complements national policies and runs for a six-year period, aims to protect human health and improve public health (European Commission, 2003). The EU also provides governance over broader issues relevant to health – for example through the EU Directive on Services (EPHA, 2005) and the Clinical Trials Directive (European Commission, 2001).

Within the UK, devolution is the main trend shaping the governance of health. There are two aspects to this. The first relates to devolution to the *home countries.* With the establishment of the Welsh Assembly and the Scottish Parliament, Wales and Scotland have the opportunity to plan and develop their own health policies on many issues, including control of (regional) NHS, community care and food safety (DH, 2000; 2002c). This has resulted in surprising levels of variation across the countries (Greer, 2004b) which will continue into the future. Devolution to English regions is also a possibility (DH, 2002c).

The second aspect of devolution concerns *'empowering the frontline'.* This is most noticeable in England, where devolution of budgetary, managerial and other responsibility to primary care trusts (PCTs) aims to transfer power from the centre to local levels of service delivery.

In England, this increased autonomy has been coupled with expansion in *regulation.* Regulation will continue to be an important component of governance but with increasing consolidation of regulators to fewer larger organisations, such as to the Healthcare Commission at present (DH, 2004f; 2004g).

Clinical governance is a major programme within the NHS focusing on the organisation's duty of quality (DH, 2000). It ensures clinical and management responsibility for systems that guarantee quality of service. This system of board and executive responsibility for the quality of clinical care has become firmly established within NHS organisations and has been adopted by private sector health organisations. It will continue to develop in the home countries and new types of health organisations in the UK.

Changes in regulation are linked to issues concerning 'modernisation', 'value for money' and public sector reform. They will continue to be important to governance as increasing public financial investments are made in the NHS (HM Treasury, 2004). It is anticipated that performance management and target-setting cultures will increasingly focus on access, quality and choice, and may become more localised.

A further discernible trend in governance is improving *patient and public engagement*. Local authorities will continue to press for more democratic engagement and responsibility for health and health organisations. The development of unitary local authorities and city boards may also increase the pressure for local authorities to take responsibility for the governance, management or regulation of health organisations (LGA *et al.*, 2004). The involvement of the private sector with the English NHS in ambulatory care, primary care and social care is likely to increase. Public/private partnerships require competent governance arrangements for stewardship of the resource and assurance of quality of care.

Trends

The following trends regarding governance and health can be identified:

- continuing, complex and uneven effects of globalisation on health, with a need for co-operative responses
- increasing direct involvement of EU institutions in public health and health protection
- rising indirect impact of EU law on domestic health policies
- continuing and increasing divergence in health policy trends in the home countries, as a result of continuing devolution
- more powers devolved to 'frontline' services (mainly in England), including PCTs
- further top-down regulation of performance, quality and value for money
- increasing emphasis on patient and public involvement in healthcare and health policy.

Current policy

The global nature of health governance is increasingly reflected through policy. This can be seen in the areas of disease control and the global labour market, as has been evident in response to SARS.

The EU too has an indirect impact on UK health policy – for example, through judgements from the European Court of Justice on whether a human being is defined as a human being from conception or from birth (European Commission, 2002a). Current policies allow for greater movement of services, staff and patients across borders. EU directives cover themes ranging from food supplements (EFSA, 2004) to bio-tech patenting (EPO, 2001). While healthcare remains within the jurisdiction of the individual countries, legislation such as the Working Time Directive has had a significant impact on the working hours of the medical staff within the NHS. Local UK services are increasingly measured against European and international peers rather than just within the NHS (University Hospital Birmingham, 2003; HM Treasury 2004).

On devolution within the UK, the plethora of policy making – measured in terms of new initiatives introduced for health – has varied between the countries. Northern Ireland has introduced policies at the slowest pace (Greer, 2004a). Wales works within current funding levels decided by the Treasury and the Scottish Parliament is able to raise or lower taxes by a maximum of three pence in the pound. Each home country has produced its own NHS and public health policy.[1] Since devolution, Scotland has abolished the internal market and is trying to increase the role of professionals. Wales has adopted localism through decentralisation and enlarged the role of local government. Northern Ireland has a weak centre, with very little policy or reorganisation (Greer, 2005). Outcomes across the four countries are increasingly uneven (Wanless, 2001).

There is myriad policy aimed at empowering frontline services in England. This has involved restructuring the NHS, increasing the role of government in regulation (corporate and clinical governance), changing funding arrangements, creating a greater role for patient and public engagement and giving greater focus to public health. Restructuring has included the formation of foundation hospitals, PCTs and strategic health authorities (DH, 2002c). In England, greater use is being made of the private sector in the delivery of care (Milburn, 1999).

NHS financial reforms were announced in *NHS Plan, Shifting the Balance of Power* and *Delivering the NHS Plan* (DH 1997; 2002a; 2002c) and have been associated with the establishment of foundation trust hospitals and increasing autonomy for primary care. Payment by results (DH 2002a; 2002b) is designed to increase transparency, efficiency, encourage quality improvements in trusts and other providers, as well as increase patient choice. This policy is still developing and so subject to change. Running alongside it is *Practice Based Commissioning* (DH, 2004e), which expands the role of individual primary care practices in commissioning. This is an evolving agenda, designed to support efficiency, empowerment of frontline staff and greater patient choice, but there are concerns about the competence of practices to commission (Nolan and Mooney, 2004).

Currently, regulation is undertaken by the Commission for Social Care Inspection and the Healthcare Commission – alongside Monitor, which inspects foundation hospitals. In a bid to reduce the burden of inspection there is a move away from targets to standards (Lloyd, 2004). NHS bodies now also have a statutory duty to ensure quality provision (DH, 2002a).

The Health and Social Care Act (2001) places a duty on NHS organisations to involve patients and the public (DH 2003b; 2004c). Patient and Public Involvement (PPI) Forums were established to monitor services and will continue to operate, although the national organising body – Commission for Patient and Public Involvement in Health (CPPIH) – will be abolished (DH, 2004f). These are expected to work closely with Local Authority Overview and Scrutiny Committees (OSCs).

Patient choice is firmly on the agenda (DH, 2003a). Current policy also gives greater involvement to the public as patients, first set out in the NHS Plan (DH, 2000). Following *Building on the Best: choice, responsiveness and equity in the NHS*

---

[1] *Putting Patients First* (Wales 1998); *Improving Health in Wales: a plan for the NHS with its partners* (2001); *Plan for the Future: a White Paper for Wales* (2001); *Investing for Health* (Northern Ireland 2002), *Partnership for Care: Scotland's Health White Paper* (2003).

consultation (DH, 2003a), the 'Choose and Book' initiative will allow patients in England to choose out of four to five providers for elective treatment (DH, 2004a). Choice is a central plank of policy for both major parties (Conservative Party, 2004; Reid, 2005).

The importance of public and individual responsibility for health can be seen in recent policy documents (Wanless, 2002; 2004; DH, 2004b; 2004d). The capacity of government to protect health, however, is less clear given the current state of the public health law and lack of clarity regarding responsibilities (Sparrow, 2005).

References

Conservative Party (2004) *Right to Choose. Health Issue.* The Conservative Party, London.

DH (1997) *The NHS Plan: a first class service.* Department of Health, London.

DH (2000) *The NHS Plan: a plan for investment, a plan for reform. Cmnd 4818–I.* The Stationery Office, London.

DH (2002a) *Delivering the NHS Plan: next steps on investment, next steps on reform.* Department of Health, London.

DH (2002b) *Reforming NHS financial flows: payment by results.* Department of Health, London.

DH (2002c) *Shifting the Balance of Power – the next steps.* Department of Health, London.

DH (2003a) *Building on the Best: choice, responsiveness and equity in the NHS.* Department of Health, London.

DH (2003b) *Strengthening accountability – involving patients and the public: policy guidance. Section 11 of the Health and Social Care Act 2001.* Department of Health, London.

DH (2004a) *Choose and Book: patient choice of hospital and booked appointment.* Department of Health, London.

DH (2004b) *Choosing Health: making healthier choices easier. Cmnd 6374.* The Stationery Office, London.

DH (2004c) *National Standards, Local Action. Health and Social Care Standards and Planning Framework 2005/06–2007/08.* Department of Health, London.

DH (2004d) *NHS Improvement Plan: putting people at the heart of public services.* Department of Health, London.

DH (2004e) *Practice Based Commissioning: engaging practices in commissioning.* Department of Health, London.

DH (2004f) *Reconfiguring the Department of Health's Arm's Length Bodies.* Department of Health, London.

DH (2004g) Standards for better health: health care standards for services under the NHS. http://www.dh.gov.uk/assetRoot/04/08/23/39/04082339.pdf. Accessed:10 February 2004.

EFSA (2004) Moving towards full strength. http://www.efsa.eu.int/about_efsa/catindex_en.html. Accessed: 1 April 2005.

EPHA (2005) Putting Citizens' Health at the Heart of Europe. http://www.epha.org/a/1317. Accessed: 1 April 2005.

EPO (2001) The strategic direction for the European Patent Office. http://www.european-patent-office.org/mit/mission_en.pdf. Accessed: 1 April 2005.

European Commission (2001) On the approximation of the laws, regulations and administrative provisions of the Member States relating to the implementation of good clinical practice in the conduct of clinical trials on medicinal products for human use. *Official Journal of the European Communities.* L 121/34: 34–44.

European Commission (2002a) 1.2.1 Parliament resolution on sexual and reproductive health and rights. Human Rights (1/7). *Bulletin of the EU.* 7/8–2002.

European Commission (2002b) Adopting a programme of community action in the field of public health (2003–2008). *Official Journal of the European Communities.* L 271/1.

European Commission (2003) Health and consumer protection (14/18). *Bulletin of the EU.* 12–2003.

Greer S (2004a) Chapter Six: Northern Ireland: permissive managerialism. In: C Jeffery (ed.) *Territorial Politics and Health Policy.* Manchester University Press, Manchester.

Greer S (2004b) *Four Way Bet: how devolution has led to four different models for the NHS.* University College London, London.

Greer S (2005) Why do good politics make bad health policy? In: S Dawson and C Sausman (eds) *Future Health Organisations and Systems.* Palgrave Macmillan, Basingstoke.

Ham C (2004) *Health Policy in Britain.* Palgrave Macmillan, Basingstoke.

HM Treasury (2004) *Value for Money Assessment Guidance.* The Stationary Office, London.

LGA, NHS Confederation and UKPHA (2004) *Public Health White Paper Misses Opportunities for Radical Improvement.* Local Government Association, London.

Lloyd I (2004) Commission chief says trusts can't treat 'health check' as a project. *Health Service Journal.* 114: 6.

Milburn A (1999) Speech by Chief Secretary to the Treasury, Alan Milburn, at the Launch of the IPPR Commission into Public/Private Partnerships. 20 September 1999. London.

Nolan A and Mooney H (2004) 'Streamlining' PCTs will shift to managing role. *Health Service Journal.* 114: 7.

Reid J (2005) *Limits of the Market, Constraints of the State: the public good and the NHS.* The Social Market Foundation, London.

Sparrow A (2005) Health Secretary denies he ignored MRSA memo. *The Telegraph.* 9.3.05.

University Hospital Birmingham (2003) *Corporate Strategy 2003–2010.* University Hospital Birmingham, Birmingham.

Wanless D (2001) *Securing our Future Health: taking a long-term view. Interim Report.* HM Treasury, London.

Wanless D (2002) *Securing our Future Health: taking a long-term view.* HM Treasury, London.

Wanless D (2004) *Securing Good Health for the Whole Population. Final Report.* HM Treasury, London.

WHO (2004) Avian influenza. Fact sheet. http://www.who.int/mediacentre/factsheets/avian_influenza/en/. Accessed: 6 April 2004.

Economics

The NHS and health sector in the UK are located within the wider national and international economy. The public share of total health expenditure in the UK is 82%, compared to an average of 72% in OECD countries (OECD, 2003). The NHS is funded principally through general taxation. It is considered important to the domestic economy because it is the largest employer in the UK.

In comparison with similar nations, the NHS has been under-resourced. Health expenditure per capita was $1989 in 2001 compared with Switzerland's $3322 and Germany's $3820 (WHO, 2004). In 2002, however, the UK Government announced an unprecedented increase of funding for the NHS. Over five years, the NHS budget will rise by 43% in real terms – an increase in real terms by an average of 7.4% for each of the next five years. In part, this is funded by a 1% increase in national insurance contributions. The total NHS budget will rise from £65.4 billion in 2002–03 to £105.6 billion in 2007–08, bringing the proportion of GDP spent on the NHS from its current level of 7.7% to 8.7% in 2005–06 and 9.4% in 2007–08. Tobacco revenues of £9.3 billion are also being directed to health in the form of a hypothecated tax.

Although there is an increase in government funding, demographic changes, an ageing population and the rise of technology put continual pressure on the NHS budget. There has been significant debate and public consultation on the sustainability of taxation as the main source of NHS finance (Wanless, 2002). Funding alternatives to taxation include medical savings accounts, a more widespread use of health insurance, increased co-payments or a combination of these measures (Adam Smith Institute, 2003; Mossialos *et al.*, 2002). Several recent reports, including the first Wanless report (2002), have concluded that alternative methods of funding may not offer significant advantages over taxation-based financing. In addition, the model of a public, national service funded from taxation performs well internationally in terms of equity and cost control (New Policy Institute, 2003).

A major push from government is expected to result in 15% of elective surgery being carried out in the private sector by the independent sector through Independent Sector Treatment Centres (ISTCs) by 2008 (DH, 2004d). More than a quarter of UK dental patients now pay privately for their dental care (Laing & Buisson, 2002a), while only 50% of general dental practitioners in the UK treat virtually all of their patients on the NHS (Laing & Buisson, 2003).

Some sectors within the UK health economy have already been significantly privatised. Of the 16 000 opticians in the UK, corporate bodies manage 60% and 40% are independently owned (Coe, 2004). The private sector is also likely to be increasingly involved in chronic disease management. Currently, 33.1% of long-term care is provided by the private sector (Laing & Buisson, 2003). Mental health is the fastest growing sector of independent healthcare, as the NHS increasingly outsources acute psychiatric care (Laing & Buisson, 2002b).

From 1996 to 2001, sales of over-the-counter drugs have increased from £1275.8 million to £1710.5 million (PAGB, 1998; 2003). Nearly 12% of the population is covered by private health insurance – an increase of 5% since 1980 (Klein, 2005).

Private institutional care grew from 175 000 places in 1985 to 650 000 places in 1998, most of which were publicly funded (Health Matters, 2000). The cost of long-term care expenditure is predicted to increase 148% in real terms between 1996 and 2031, to meet demographic pressures and allow for real rises in care costs of 1% per year and 1.5% per year for healthcare (Wittenberg *et al.*, 2001). To keep pace with demographic pressures over the next 30 years, the number of residential and nursing home places will need to expand by around 65%, and numbers of home-care recipients by around 48% (Wittenberg *et al.*, 2001). This base projection assumes no changes in the health of older people. It is estimated that 7% of long-term care is provided by informal carers (Andalo, 2004).

The private sector is also growing in importance in terms of capital funding. Project Financing in England through the Private Finance Initiative (PFI) allows private sector consortia to fund hospital building programmes. PFI has been extended to primary care through the LIFT programmes (Local Improvement Finance Trust) (DH, 2004b) and is likely to continue as a method of injecting capital into the NHS – although it is not used in Wales, Scotland or Northern Ireland.

Incentives within the NHS are changing continuously. Examples include the introduction of payment by results (PBR) for healthcare providers and new incentives in remuneration for the medical profession both in primary and hospital care to encourage medical behaviour and service patterns aligned with the NHS in the 21st Century (DH, 2004a; 2004c). The economics of the organisation are also changing as it moves from 'command and control' system hierarchies to devolved networks, such as cancer networks, and devolved entities, such as foundation trusts.

Trends

Some trends that become apparent are:

- increased funding and resource levels throughout the NHS
- relatively low privatisation of financing, but increases in private project financing and the delivery of health services
- increased involvement of the private sector in the English NHS in the provision of elective care and chronic disease management
- changing economic incentives in UK health and move to devolved structures
- increasing interdependence between the NHS and the health economy and the wider economies of the home countries and the UK as a whole.

Current policy

Increased reliance on individual responsibility may shift the financial burden of the patient away from the 'traditional' NHS. There may be a renegotiation of the social contract, whereby citizens could pay more for services.

The government in England has an explicit policy of maintaining tax-based funding for the NHS and encouraging plurality and diversity of provision (DH, 2004b; Milburn, 2003; Reid, 2005). The involvement of the private sector in the NHS is an explicit policy option chosen by the current government to address some of the deficiencies of the NHS. Measures introduced include: the encouragement of NHS organisations to form joint ventures with the private or voluntary sector under Public Private Partnerships (PPP);[2] the creation of Independent Sector Treatment

---

[2] Public Private Partnerships (PPP) is the umbrella name given to a range of initiatives which involve the private sector in the operation of public services. The Private Finance Initiative (PFI) is the most frequently used initiative. The key difference between PFI and conventional ways of providing public services is that the public does not own the asset. The authority makes an annual payment to the private company who provides the building and associated services, rather like a mortgage.

Centres for ambulatory surgery and other care; encouraging a diversity of private and not-for-profit providers to compete for NHS contracts for secondary care; and a greater choice of health service providers for patients. Patients whose needs may not be met by the NHS are able to seek care (and be reimbursed by the NHS) either abroad within the EU or in the private sector (DH, 2002).

Devolution of budgetary control for primary and secondary care to the Primary Care Trusts (PCTs) shifts the responsibility of resource allocation further, to the local level. From April 2005, GPs have been given more control of their budgets currently with PCTs. It is believed that this commissioning of services will lead to fewer hospital admissions as GPs may be more responsive to patient needs (DH, 2004d; 2004e). PCTs are sometimes unwilling to hand over their budgets, however, and not all GPs are enthusiastic about practice-based commissioning (BBC News, 2005).

Future economic pressures include increasing workforce costs and demands for new technology. The government has committed to raise staffing and resource levels throughout the Health Service, for example through a 30% increase in medical school intake. More recruitment of foreign clinical staff and focus on private-sector involvement may be anticipated if the government intends to achieve its challenging goals.

The injection of market forces into the NHS continues to be the subject of intense debate and controversy. The government argues that private-sector initiatives are more cost-effective, efficient and better run than public bodies, and that the private sector offers much-needed capital to the NHS. Private sector finance and management added about 40% to the total cost of each project (Pollock, 2004), however, and the impact of greater plurality on quality and outcomes has yet to be established (Dixon, *et al.*, 2003). In England, the government is introducing a payment-by-result system that reimburses hospitals on a fixed-tariff basis for specified procedures of care (DH, 2004c; DH *et al.*, 2003). Coupled with patient choice, this will mean that a hospital's income depends on whether patients wish to be treated there (Taylor, 2005).

An important backdrop to current policies on the future of the NHS is the increasing role of agencies such as the Healthcare Commission, NICE and the Modernisation Agency and their counterparts in Wales, Scotland and Northern Ireland (*see* Governance on page 28). In 2002, it became mandatory for PCTs to implement NICE guidance, lending organisations further authority. The government is discussing the issue of rationing within the health service more openly, recognising that with increased treatments and increased potential for treatment, there needs to be more clarity over what the health service funds and what it does not. The importance of evidence-based medicine, health technology assessment, rigorous scrutiny of the economic and clinical value of new technologies and the standardisation of treatment protocols remain driving trends within the NHS. There has also been a significant investment of £2.3 billion in IT infrastructure (Caldwell, 2003). A tightened regulatory environment is intended to drive the efficiency and quality of health service provision throughout the NHS.

References

Adam Smith Institute (2003) Medical savings accounts – could medical savings accounts provide the escape from runaway healthcare costs? http://www.adamsmith.org/cissues/medical-savings-account.htm. Accessed: 16 March 2004.

Andalo D (2004) Elderly care costs 'to increase'. *The Guardian*. 7.5.04.

BBC News (2005) Many GPs 'snubbing NHS changes'. http://news.bbc.co.uk/1/hi/health/4359497.stm. Accessed: 25 March 2005.

Caldwell K (2003) The National Programme for Information Technology in the NHS in England (NPfIT). http://www.hisi.ie/html/ppt03/Kevin%20Caldwell%20NHS%20IT.pdf. Accessed: 25 March 2004.

Coe P (2004) Personal communication. Email to: Chang, L.

DH (2002) *Delivering the NHS Plan: next steps on investment, next steps on reform*. Department of Health, London.

DH (2004a) *Delivering the HR in the NHS Plan 2004*. Department of Health, London.

DH (2004b) *Guidance on the use of enabling funds: ENABLING FUNDS FOR LIFT*. Department of Health, London.

DH (2004c) *National tariff 2005–06*. Department of Health, London.

DH (2004d) *NHS Improvement Plan: putting people at the heart of public services*. Department of Health, London.

DH (2004e) *Practice Based Commissioning: engaging practices in commissioning*. Department of Health, London.

DH, NHS Modernisation Agency and National Primary and Care Trust Development Team (NatPaCT) (2003) *Reforming NHS Financial Flows: introducing payment by results*. Department of Health, London.

Dixon J, LeGrand J and Smith P (2003) *Can Market Forces be Used for Good?* King's Fund, London.

Health Matters (2000) Globalisation? Privatisation! *Health Matters*. **41**.

Klein R (2005) The public-private mix in the UK. In: A Maynard (ed.) *The Public-Private Mix for Health*. Radcliffe Publishing, Oxford, pp. 41–60.

Laing & Buisson (2002a) *Dentistry*. Laing & Buisson, London.

Laing & Buisson (2002b) *Thriving Private Hospital Market*. Laing & Buisson, London.

Laing & Buisson (2003) *Long-term Care: value of the care home market*. Laing & Buisson, London.

Milburn A (2003) Full text: Alan Milburn's speech. *The Guardian*. 5.3.03.

Mossialos E, Dixon A, Figueras J and Kulzin J (2002) *Funding Health Care: options for Europe*. European Observatory on Healthcare Systems, Buckingham.

New Policy Institute (2003) Monitoring Poverty and Social Exclusion. Key Facts. http://www.poverty.org.uk/summary/key_facts.htm. Accessed: 17 March 2004.

OECD (2003) *Health at a Glance. OECD Indicators 2003*. Organisation for Economic Cooperation and Development, Paris.

PAGB (1998) *Annual Report 1998*. The Proprietary Association of Great Britain, London.

PAGB (2003) *Annual Report 2002*. The Proprietary Association of Great Britain, London.

Pollock AM (2004) *NHS Plc: the privatisation of our health care*. Verso, London.

Reid J (2005) *Limits of the Market, Constraints of the State: the public good and the NHS*. The Social Market Foundation, London.

Taylor R (2005) Variations in waiting times: data briefing. *Health Service Journal*. **115**: 25.

Wanless D (2002) *Securing our Future Health: taking a long-term view*. HM Treasury, London.

WHO (2004) Countries. http://www.who.int/country/en/. Accessed: 16 March 2004.

Wittenberg R, Pickard L, Comas-Herrera A, Davies B and Darton R (2001) Demand for long-term care for old people in England to 2031. *Health Statistics Quarterly*. **12**: 5.

Industry

Industry, or the private sector, is playing an increasingly important role in shaping the provision of healthcare and health policy in the UK. Broadly defined, industry encompasses private providers of health and social services (sometimes paid for with public money), private health insurance and alternative therapies. Manufacturers and distributors of medical devices and pharmaceutical products are important to the health industry, which is growing. It is increasingly consolidated through mergers and acquisitions (Gershon, 2000), makes great use of outsourcing (Crossley, 2004) and is subject to increased scrutiny for corporate governance and accountability.

Private sector involvement, in partnership with the NHS, in the delivery of care and systems for the management of chronic disease is likely to increase (DH, 2004a). With the ageing of the population, private and voluntary sector social services, long-term care and home-care service providers are interacting increasingly with 'classic' NHS providers. These changes are modifying the traditional delivery and organisation of healthcare and encouraging close collaboration between complementary services regarding the patient. Private health insurance accounts for 12% of healthcare expenditure in the UK and is likely to remain at this level in future. Practitioners of alternative and complementary medicine are becoming more pervasive and more regulated (Dixon *et al.*, 2003). More than half of GPs now recommend alternative therapies to patients (*The Economist,* 2004).

According to the Department of Trade and Industry (DTI) (2003), the UK currently has the largest biotechnology industry in Europe. The *bioscience/healthcare sector*, which encompasses diagnostic, device, service and supply companies – but excludes major pharmaceutical companies – includes over 1100 companies, employs 100 000 people and generates revenues of £11 billion.

The main industry player is still the *pharmaceutical industry*, which employs close to 70 000 people in the UK and invests over £9 million daily in research and development (R&D) (ABPI, 2005). The UK plays an important role in global drug discovery, with more than a quarter of the world's top 100 medicines being developed in laboratories in Britain (ABPI, 2005).

Technology is likely to contribute to better health in future. Pharmacogenetics, in particular, yields promise for the development of 'tailored therapies' and genetic screening. These may significantly alter the uptake of medicines and future approaches to care, adding a layer of complexity to the regulatory guidelines and principles currently in place, as well as impacting on costs.

Three concurrent trends presently affect the pharmaceutical industry in the UK. First, the costs of *research and development (R&D)* are rising, with progressively lower yields in terms of new drugs reaching the market. Recognising this risk, government and industry are joining forces to foster investment in R&D, and to increase the competitiveness and productivity of the pharmaceutical industry in the UK and Europe. The Pharmaceutical Industry Competitiveness Task Force (PICTF) was set up to identify steps to retain and strengthen the UK as an attractive business environment for an innovative pharmaceutical industry. PICTF addressed a broad range of issues relevant to the industry and its relationship with government, regulators and the NHS (ABPI, 2005). A key recommendation was that clinical trials of drugs with no overtly commercial aims can now be financed through joint funding from the NHS and the commercial sector.

Second, industry is subject to increased *scrutiny* in terms of its overall ethical role as a purveyor of medicines on the NHS. A seminal report by the King's Fund states that the relationship between the pharmaceutical industry and the government should be driven by 'the promotion of health, not just the promotion of wealth' (Harrison, 2003). The same document urges pharmaceutical companies to direct their research where it is most needed, as opposed to where greatest profits could be derived (Harrison, 2003). There is a recognised need to use publicly-funded investment in research and tax incentives so as to direct pharmaceuticals and health services research towards socially beneficial health targets that run the risk of not being met because they are not economically attractive (BBC, 2002; DTI, 2003). At the European level, a proposal to legalise direct-to-consumer advertising by pharmaceutical companies was rejected by the European Parliament, on the grounds that the risks of false advertising to doctors and patients were far too high (Villanueva *et al.*, 2003).

The third trend relates to *cost-containment*. Pharmaceutical expenditure in the NHS is low compared to other EU countries, despite relatively high drug prices. Nonetheless, the rapid pace of technological advancement and the introduction of newer, expensive medicines cause this expenditure to grow year by year. The significant expansion of existing drugs budgets will be needed to meet the government objectives of service provision and to comply with NICE guidance, namely regarding the provision of statins to cardiac patients (Heart Protection Study Collaborative Group, 2003).

For this reason, increased attention is being given to Health Technology Assessment (HTA), or the evaluation of the economic and clinical value of new technologies, to determine the 'added value' and cost-effectiveness of new medicines being introduced within the NHS. The House of Commons is currently undertaking an Inquiry on new technologies (House of Commons Health Committee, 2004a). The role and value of NICE, created in 1999, was the subject of intense debate in 2002–04. The House of Commons Health Select Committee conducted a review of NICE and called for a further independent, peer assessment of the Institute's work (House of Commons Health Select Committee, 2002). The latter was undertaken by WHO (Hill *et al.*, 2003). Both reports, although critical in some respects, reinforced the importance of the Institute's work for the NHS.

Trends

Some trends regarding health and industry include:

- increasing use of the private sector in health and social care provision
- increasing recognition of the important economic role of the bioscience/ healthcare sector
- increasing collaboration between the pharmaceutical industry and government to stimulate scientific advance and innovation
- increasing R&D costs associated with bioscience and a growing focus on health technology assessments to guide resource allocation decisions
- continuing attempts to contain NHS costs.

Current policy

The UK government is strongly advocating further involvement of the private sector, and all sectors of industry, with the NHS. In England, there is a clear policy trend towards significant involvement of the private sector in provision of health-care and social care.

Various policy documents issued since 2003 suggest greater co-operation and partnership between the NHS, universities and industry (HM Treasury, 2003; Research for Patient Benefit Working Party (RPBWP) 2004). They recognise that the NHS provides a unique source for clinical trials and could steer the direction of research more forcefully (Harrison, 2003). The government is playing a role in pushing the pharmaceutical industry to develop drugs in areas of most unmet medical need, particularly with the Treasury's recent announcement of tax incentives for companies that conduct research into 'neglected' diseases (Inland Revenue, 2005). Changes to the Pharmaceutical Price Regulation Scheme are also designed to support a 'competitive' industry (DH, 2005).

There is increasing recognition of the crucial economic role played by the UK health technology industry (DTI, 2003; HITF, 2004a,b) and the need for policy to support development. Funding in science has recently increased. The UK plans to spend an extra £1 billion on science by 2008 (HM Treasury *et al.*, 2004), which is double the expenditure on science in 1997.

The government plans to take a more active role in developing some aspects of technology. *Our Inheritance, Our Future: realising the potential of genetics in the NHS* sets out plans to develop genetic services (DH, 2003a) and was followed by an announcement of £18 million being made available to upgrade genetics laboratories (10 Downing Street, 2004). The Human Genetics Commission (HGC) has consulted over a range of controversial issues, including the creation of siblings for treatment of existing children and will report to Ministers later in 2005 (HGC, 2004).

Public perceptions have a strong influence on regulation, and a supportive regulatory environment in the UK and Europe is critical to the success of the UK bioscience and pharmaceutical sectors. The outcome of the current House of Commons Health Committee Review of the Pharmaceutical Industry (2004b) will have far-reaching implications: the challenge is to maintain a manageable system of regulation, striking a balance between protecting people from harm and supporting innovation. Getting the balance wrong could result in significant costs to public health, and may imperil the competitiveness of the UK's bioscience industry.

Regulatory bodies relevant to the healthcare industry have been reorganised as a result of the Department of Health's Review of Arm's Length Bodies (DH, 2004b). The Human Fertilisation and Embryology Authority and the proposed Human Tissue Authority have merged to form the Regulatory Authority for Fertility and Tissue (RAFT). The Review also proposes that the Central Office for Research Ethics Committee be incorporated into the National Patient Safety Agency. The Medicines and Healthcare Products Regulatory Agency (MHRA), which resulted from the merger of the Medicines Control Agency and the Medical Devices Agency in April 2003, is responsible for regulating the handling and preparation of medicinal products, as well as applications for their use in clinical trials.

Increasingly, the primary forum for regulatory debates is Europe, and it is important for the UK to play a leading role (DTI, 2003). Some academics are already suggesting that the EU Clinical Trials Directive introduced in May 2004 will render their small-scale trials impossibly expensive as a result of science shifting elsewhere (Tomlinson, 2004). The issues of patents, generic drugs and price controls remain central as the government struggles between conflicting roles: stimulating innovation and economic growth while at the same time curtailing health expenditure.

The pharmaceutical and medical devices industry is strongly affected by globalisation and EU policy, particularly in terms of increasing cross-border flows of people, goods, services and capital. What is exceptional with medicines is that they are considered 'goods and services' within the EU context, and therefore subject to free movement across different country borders. But individual countries have control and governance over deciding whether a drug should be reimbursed and at what price it should be sold within its national healthcare market. However, it is completely legal for parallel importers to import or export drugs between member states within the EU, playing on the differences in prices between countries. This is an important issue limiting the competitiveness of the pharmaceutical market in Europe (compared to, for example, the US). In a recent study by Kanavos *et al.* (2004), it was shown that national healthcare systems and patients gained little from drugs being made available at lower prices because most of the profits were pocketed by the parallel importers. The expansion of the EU in May 2004 also has significant implications for the migration of health workers and patients, as well as parallel distribution of pharmaceuticals within the EU.

Overall, government policy continues to be affected by economic and cost-containment demands within the NHS. While industrial policy aims to develop stronger links between stakeholders, Health Technology Assessment continues to be a major policy tool. In October 2001, for example, NICE decisions became mandatory and in 2004 an 'Implementation Tsar' (Freemantle, 2004) was appointed to aid this process. From an industry perspective the issue is the extent to which NICE acts as a bottleneck or barrier. NICE did not approve atypical anti-psychotics until 2002, for example, which was ten years after they had entered clinical practice.

A series of policies relate to deregulating pharmaceutical services. *Pharmacy in the Future: implementing the NHS Plan* (DH, 2000) set out the government's plans for expanding the role of pharmacists and was followed by *A Vision for Pharmacy in the New NHS* (DH, 2003b). These aim to make greater use of community pharmacists in delivering primary care and public health services.

References

10 Downing Street (2004) £18m genetics boost for England. http://www.number-10.gov.uk/output/Page6066.asp. Accessed: 29 March 2005.

ABPI (2005) The Association of the British Pharmaceutical Industry. http://www.abpi.org.uk/. Accessed: 30 March 2005.

BBC (2002) Deal promises new drugs. BBC News. 25.03.02. BBC, London.

Crossley R (2004) The quiet revolution: outsourcing in pharma. *Drug Discovery Today.* 9(16): 694.

DH (2000) *Pharmacy in the Future: Implementing the NHS Plan: a programme for pharmacy in the National Health Service.* Department of Health, London.

DH (2003a) *Our Inheritance, Our Future: realising the potential of genetics in the NHS. Cmnd 5791–II.* Department of Health, London.

DH (2003b) *A Vision for Pharmacy in the NHS*. TSO, London.

DH (2004a) *NHS Improvement Plan: putting people at the heart of public services*. Department of Health, London.

DH (2004b) *Reconfiguring the Department of Health's Arm's Length Bodies*. Department of Health, London.

DH (2005) Pharmaceutical Price Regulation Scheme. http://www.dh.gov.uk/PolicyAndGuidance/MedicinesPharmacyAndIndustry/PharmaceuticalPriceRegulationScheme/fs/en. Accessed: 29 March 2005.

Dixon A, Saka O, Le Grand J, Riesberg A, Weinbrenner S and Busse R (2003) *Complementary and Alternative Medicine in the UK and Germany – research and evidence on supply and demand*. Anglo-German Foundation for the Study of Industrial Society, London.

DTI (2003) *Bioscience 2015. Improving National Health, Increasing National Wealth*. Department of Trade and Industry, Bioscience Innovation and Growth Team, London.

Freemantle N (2004) Commentary: Is NICE delivering the goods? *British Medical Journal*. **329**: 1003–4.

Gershon D (2000) Are mega-mergers good medicine for the pharmaceutical industry? *Nature*. **405**: 257–8.

Harrison A (2003) *Getting the right medicines? Putting public interests at the heart of health-related research (Summary)*. King's Fund, London.

Heart Protection Study Collaborative Group (2003) MRC/BHF Heart Protection Study of cholesterol-lowering with simvastatin in 5963 people with diabetes: a randomised placebo-controlled trial. *The Lancet*. **361**(9375): 2005–16.

HGC (2004) *Human Genetics Commission Consultation, Choosing the Future: genetics and reproductive decision making*. Human Genetics Commission, London.

Hill S, Garattini S, Loenhout JV, O'Brian BJ and Joncheere KD (2003) *Technology Appraisal Programme of the National Institute for Clinical Excellence*. World Health Organization, London.

HITF (2004a) *HITF Working Group 2 R&D and the Industrial Base Little Working Group – a few 'big hits'*. Healthcare Industries Task Force, London.

HITF (2004b) *Reports from Working Groups and Overview of Key Recommendations (Draft)*. Healthcare Industries Task Force, London.

HM Treasury (2003) *Lambert Review of Business–University Collaboration. Final Report*. HM Treasury, London.

HM Treasury, Department of Trade and Industry and Department of Education and Skills (2004) *Science & Innovation Investment Framework 2004–2014*. HM Treasury, London.

House of Commons Health Committee (2004a) New Inquiry: the use of new medical technologies within the NHS. http://www.parliament.uk/parliamentary_committees/health_committee/hc071204_03.cfm. Accessed: 30 March 2005.

House of Commons Health Committee (2004b) New Inquiry: the influence of the pharmaceutical industry: health policy, research, prescribing practice and patient use. http://www.parliament.uk/parliamentary_committees/health_committee/hc180604_25.cfm. Accessed: 30 March 2005.

House of Commons Health Select Committee (2002) *House of Commons Health Committee, Second Report of Session 2001–02*. House of Commons, London.

Inland Revenue (2005) REV 2: A Competitive and Modern Tax System for Multi-Nationals and Large Business. http://www.inlandrevenue.gov.uk/budget2001/rev2.htm. Accessed: 29 March 2005.

Kanavos P, Costa-I-Font J, Merkur S and Gemmill M (2004) *The Economic Impact of Pharmaceutical Parallel Trade in European Union Member States: a stakeholder analysis. Special Research Paper. LSE. Health and Social Care*. London School of Economics, London.

Research for Patient Benefit Working Party (RPBWP) (2004) *Final Report*. Department of Health, London.

The Economist (2004) Quacks Unite! *The Economist*. 6 March 2004, pp. 30–1.

Tomlinson H (2004) Medical research 'stifled by rules'. *The Guardian*. 6.12.04.

Villanueva P, Peiró S, Librero J and Pereiró I (2003) The accuracy of pharmaceutical advertisement in medical journals. *The Lancet*. **361**(9351): 27–31.

Chapter 2

Legal context

Sheila McLean

Despite its all-pervasiveness in society, the role of the law in health, healthcare and wellbeing is sometimes underestimated. Contemporary attention tends to focus instead on ethics or to conflate the two. People are generally familiar with statutes impacting directly on wellbeing, such as mental health legislation, but the common law and international agreements are directly relevant forms of law too. In its widest sense, law has a profound impact on health, wellbeing and healthcare. This chapter concentrates on the issues deemed most likely to inform the health policy process in the next 15 years. These are:

- the Human Rights Act 1998
- the changing 'contract' between providers of healthcare and patients
- redress.

The final sections of the chapter consider key issues relating to:

- technology
- globalisation.

The Human Rights Act 1998

The significance of international norms for the domestic agenda is most clearly highlighted by the incorporation into UK law of the Council of Europe's Convention on Human Rights by the Human Rights Act 1998. Since incorporation, all legislation passed by the UK parliaments must be certified as compatible with the Convention, courts must take account of the Convention-based jurisprudence and individuals can raise human rights issues directly in UK courts.

In the future, the statutory protection of certain human rights will have implications for the health and wellbeing of UK citizens. The meanings to be given to Article 2 (the right to life), Article 3 (no one shall be subjected to torture or to inhuman or degrading treatment or punishment) and Article 8 (the right to private and family life), for example, have already been the subject of litigation on a number of occasions. In some ways these cases have perpetuated existing legal positions – for example, *Osman v United Kingdom*[1] confirmed that the state's positive obligation to preserve life, under Article 2, is not absolute and that issues such as resources and clinical diagnosis are also relevant.[2] The recent case of *David Glass v The United Kingdom*[3] also adjudicated on issues involving Article 6 (the right to a fair

---

[1] (1999) 29 HRR 245.
[2] [McLean, 2003 #982].
[3] [2004] Lloyd's Rep Med 76 (ECHR).

hearing), Article 8 (the right to private and family life), Article 13 (the right to an effective remedy) and Article 14 (the non-discrimination provision). Indirectly, human rights considerations have affected, and will continue to affect, the rights of individuals to register complaints (specifically in the case of resource allocation decisions) and to seek to vindicate their claims to a right to receive particular treatments or to refuse them. Decisions about the provision of social care have also been scrutinised from a rights-based analysis. Article 5 (the right to liberty and security of the person) will directly affect the detention provisions of mental health legislation.[4]

Most recently, in the case of *R (Burke) v General Medical Council*,[5] the right of a person to insist on receiving assisted nutrition and hydration at the end of his life, irrespective of the views of his doctors, was accepted. Although the court accepted that it would not 'grant a mandatory order requiring an individual doctor to treat a patient', it was also said that 'this does not mean that a doctor can simply decline to go on treating his patient merely because his views as to what is in his patient's best interests differ from that of the patient or the court. We no longer equate a patient's best interests as being in all circumstances what his doctor believes to be in his best interests.'[6]

Although this case seems likely to be appealed, it is significant for two main reasons. First, as is considered in more depth below, it reinforces the 'consumer-led' trend in healthcare. Whereas it would have been plausible to deduce from previous jurisprudence that courts would never (or virtually never) gainsay the clinical decision of doctors about when to offer treatment,[7] in this case the patient's choice became paramount. Second, Mr Justice Munby in the *Burke* case also specifically rejected the views of Dame Elizabeth Butler-Sloss in the case of *NHS Trust A v M, NHS Trust B v H*[8] as to the applicability of Article 3 of the Convention on Human Rights to the withdrawal of treatment from a patient in a permanent vegetative state. Butler-Sloss had argued that for Article 3 of the Convention to be engaged, the person who was allegedly receiving inhumane or degrading treatment had to be able to experience it: otherwise there was no breach of the Convention right. Mr Justice Munby, however, argued that 'treatment which has the effect on those who witness it of degrading the individual may come within Article 3. Otherwise ... the Convention's emphasis on the protection of the vulnerable may be circumvented.'[9]

Although the impact of the Human Rights Act has yet to be fully experienced in the UK, there is good reason to believe that it will have a significant impact over the next 15 years, as the traditional approach of UK courts is subject to the scrutiny of Strasbourg jurisprudence within the UK court system itself. Thus, although the Court of Human Rights in Strasbourg has been reluctant to intervene directly in matters that fall within the margin of appreciation, which allows states to maintain certain principled positions,[10] UK courts themselves may be radical in their interpretation of the Convention and its implications. As will be seen below, this will

---

[4] *Winterwerp v Netherlands* (1979) 2 EHRR 387.
[5] [2004] EWHC 1879 (Admin).
[6] para 191.
[7] *See*, for example, the case of *Re C (a minor) (medical treatment)* (1997) 40 BMLR 31; *A NHS Trust v D* (2000) 55 BMLR 19; *Re J (a minor) (wardship: medical treatment)* (1992) 9 BMLR 10.
[8] [2001] 1 All ER 801.
[9] para 145.
[10] *See*, for example, the case of *Pretty v UK* (2002) 66 BMLR 147.

also have an impact on the capacity of individual citizens to redress grievances against healthcare and other providers whose services are important to health and wellbeing.

Contracts between providers and patients

At the micro level, the relationship between the individual and deliverers of services has traditionally been rooted in the common law of negligence, which evaluates behaviour on the basis of the duty of the deliverer of the service, rather than on the rights of the recipient. Challenges were based on a vision of certain social or professional relationships as being loosely able to be described as fiduciary, or based on trust. Despite the dominance of autonomy in modern legal and ethical thinking, the common law has arguably been slow to accommodate its ramifications when professional behaviour is challenged, despite paying lip service to it. Perhaps paradoxically, however, the autonomy-based claims of individuals may lead to a sea-change in the law's approach. This is already established in consumer protection and data protection legislation, for example, and to an extent in the Freedom of Information Act 2000, where the interests (or claims, or rights) of individuals dominate the legal regime. If the common law follows suit, as is plausible to argue it will given the increasing importance attached to autonomy and now to human rights, dispute resolution will become more contractual or quasi-contractual in nature. In the future, emphasising rights will change the relationship between the individual and the state as provider of healthcare and social services, requiring it to be seen more as a quasi-contractual one based on explicit promises. Most significantly, Article 8 of the Convention on Human Rights (the right to private and family life) incorporates the equivalent of an autonomy right directly into the considerations both of legislators and courts throughout the UK.

The impact of this on the legal approach to healthcare delivery is likely to be significant. Most specifically, it will affect the way in which disputes are generated and resolved. The primary emphasis will be on the rights of the individual rather than on the duties of the state or its representatives, mandating a different analysis of the issues under consideration and challenging the current emphasis on 'professionalism' as the primary basis for judging the quality of a service. Outcome which is generated, and perhaps defined, by the expectations of the recipient of services will play a significant role in mediating disputes in the future. An apparent promise to provide healthcare resources may come to be seen as a promise to provide services necessary to the individual, rendering resource allocation or rationing decisions more difficult to justify.[11] Whether this move is to be welcomed must be the subject of informed debate.

Redress – consumer rights and autonomy

The fundamental nature of the relationship between the state and the individual is superimposed on, and sometimes drives, legal engagement in health and wellbeing. This is a special relationship in the UK because the majority of healthcare is provided

---

[11] *See*, for example, *R v Gloucestershire County Council, ex p Barry* (1997) 36 BMLR 69.

by the state. Although the rights which now form part of the UK's written law are arguably not new, their direct enforceability seems likely to reinforce the dominance of certain ethical and legal principles, most notably that of autonomy. Autonomy or self-governance has a long history as a precept but has become the driving force in law, particularly since the Nuremberg Trials. It is central to declarations and guidelines drawn up by organisations such as the United Nations, the Council of Europe, the World Medical Association and many more governmental and non-governmental organisations.

The value of autonomy has, therefore, informed legal development and regulation and has served to trump other interests in numerous situations. It is this concept that has driven the agenda of recent inquiries into medical practices, such as those into the unauthorised removal and retention of organs and tissue at post-mortem examination, and has mandated major changes to complaints mechanisms in healthcare. The emphasis on the individual as active participant rather than passive recipient of the delivery of healthcare, and on the individual as a major driver of public sector provision, has arguably redesigned the relationship between the state and the citizen. Focusing on individual rights rather than the duties of service providers has the (possibly desirable) effect of locating power with the individual. It also, however, may have the (arguably undesirable) effect of atomising individuals and separating them from the interests of others. As Callahan (1984) says; 'It [autonomy] buys our freedom to be ourselves, and to be free of undue influence by others, at too high a price ... It elevates isolation and separation ... It will inevitably diminish the sense of obligation that others may feel toward us, and shrivel our sense of obligation toward others.'[12]

Yet, the concept of autonomy is regularly raised in debates about euthanasia, reproductive liberty and many other areas that affect both health and general wellbeing. At the same time, the genetics 'revolution' informs us about what we share rather than how we are different, postulating foreseeable tensions with the predominant ethic of autonomy. It is this tension – and how it is resolved – that will be of most significance to the healthcare of the future.

Given an increased emphasis on individual rights, the common law will play an increasingly significant role in scrutinising decisions of service providers using the mechanism of judicial review.[13] This may be argued on three grounds: illegality, irrationality and 'procedural impropriety'.[14] As Palmer says, 'the purpose of judicial

---

[12] Callahan D (1984) Autonomy: a moral good, not a moral obsession. *Hastings Center Report.* **40**.

[13] Judicial review is a form of court proceeding in which a judge reviews the lawfulness of a decision or action made by a public body. It is a challenge to the *way in which a decision has been made*. It is not really concerned with the conclusions of that process and whether those were 'correct', as long as the correct procedures have been followed. The court will not substitute what it thinks is the 'correct' decision. This may mean that the public body will be able to make the same decision again, so long as it does so in a lawful way. (*See* http://www.publiclawproject.org.uk/simpleguide.html#1).

[14] By 'illegality' as a ground for judicial review the author means that the decision-maker must understand correctly the law that regulates his decision-making power and must give effect to it ... By 'irrationality' the author means what can by now be succinctly referred to as 'Wednesbury unreasonableness' (*see Associated Provincial Picture Houses Ltd v Wednesbury Corp* [1947] 2 All ER 680, [1948] 1 KB 223). It applies to a decision which is so outrageous in its defiance of logic or of accepted moral standards that no sensible person who had applied his mind to the question to be decided could have arrived at it. Whether a decision falls within this category is a question

review is the control of discretion in accordance with the rule of law',[15] and it has arguably been rendered more accessible to an aggrieved individual following the decision of the Court of Human Rights in the case of *Smith and Grady v The UK*.[16] In this case, the Court of Human Rights argued that the test traditionally employed in UK law to evaluate the decision of public authorities was too difficult to achieve.

In the short term, there may be only a limited impact following legal development in this area. It has been said that: 'Although there have been successful challenges to healthcare allocation decisions, these cases tend to turn on very specific factual situations and offer little encouragement for those who would like to see the courts take a more proactive role in the field.'[17]

The combination of attention to human rights and the decision in *Smith and Grady*, however, seems virtually certain to impact on those delivering services, not only to ensure that their decisions are 'reasonable', but also that they are procedurally correct. Thus: 'The existence of a rights discourse within a legal tradition adds an important dimension to the ... equation. It reduces the constraints imposed by traditional conceptions of judicial review and permits resource allocation questions to be conceptualised as issues of rights, rather than those of policy choice. A rights tradition permits the courts to apply their own expertise about law and rights to policy questions, rather than having to defer to the policy expertise of administrators.'[18]

Perhaps most importantly, given that resources seem unlikely ever to be able to meet demand, a transparent and principled approach needs to be taken. As Mason, McCall Smith and Laurie[19] say: 'It is inevitable that, so long as there is a restriction on resources – and there must be a limit even in Utopia – some principle of maximum societal benefit must be applied: the individual's right to equality must, to some extent, be sacrificed to the general need. The precise determination of a maximum benefit policy is difficult to make, but the decision is societal rather than medical and involves a 'cost-benefit' analysis.'[20]

---

that judges by their training and experience should be well equipped to answer, or else there would be something badly wrong with our judicial system ... the author has described the third head as 'procedural impropriety', rather than failure to observe basic rules of natural justice or failure to act with procedural fairness towards the person who will be affected by the decision. This is because susceptibility to judicial review under this head covers also failure by an administrative tribunal to observe procedural rules that are expressly laid down in the legislative instrument by which its jurisdiction is conferred, even where such failure does not involve any denial of natural justice, per Lord Diplock in *Council of Civil Service Unions v Minister for the Civil Service* (The GCHQ Case) [1985] AC 374, at p. 410 D.

[15] Palmer E (2000) Resource allocation, welfare rights – mapping the boundaries of judicial control in public administrative law. *Oxford Journal of Legal Studies.* **20**(1): 63 at p. 70.

[16] (2002) 29 EHRR 493.

[17] Sheldrick BM (2003) Judicial review and the allocation of healthcare resources in Canada and the United Kingdom. *Journal of Comparative Policy Analysis: research and practice.* **5**: 149 at p. 155.

[18] p. 157.

[19] Mason JK, McCall Smith RA and Laurie GT (2002) *Law and Medical Ethics* (6 edn). Butterworths, London.

[20] at p. 368.

Technology

Advances in technology will also directly impact on the relationship between individuals and service providers. Issues pertaining to information and genetics are discussed in more detail below.

Information

Delivery of services following the increased use of technology will significantly modify the historical power imbalance between provider and recipient. People are increasingly computer literate, which allows them to negotiate rather than simply receive services from a knowledge base, and the potential to use ID cards to store more than simple identification information, coupled with the drive towards patient-held records, will further reinforce a shift in power towards the 'consumer'. On the other hand, Gostin points to the fact that, although modern systems for storing and handling information have great benefits for research and possibly the treatment of genetic conditions, they also pose threats to privacy because of their capacity to 'store and decipher unimaginable quantities of highly sensitive data'.[21]

Individual concerns about the safety of storage and management of personal information seem likely to mean that these issues will become increasingly important. 'Consumers' are likely to demand more respect for personal information in terms of Article 8. In the case of *Chare nee Jullien v France*,[22] the Commission on Human Rights found that the collection of medical data and the maintenance of medical records fell within the sphere of private life in Article 8. Additionally, the case of *Z v Finland*[23] held that domestic law must provide appropriate standards to prevent communication or disclosure of personal health data that is inconsistent with the guarantees in Article 8. In the future the notion of partnership between the individual and the service provider will be reinforced – dictating a shift in the balance of power and reinforcing the concept of professional interventions as negotiated arrangements couched in terms of promise of outcome – but there are still issues that need to be resolved.

Genetics

Although the legal relationship between individual and the state will become increasingly focused on respect of individuals, the so-called genetics revolution has the capacity to show us how similar we are rather than how different. This may enhance the role of communities and potentially set them in competition with individual claims or interests. For instance, if it is shown to be cost-effective, or otherwise socially beneficial, to screen asymptomatic individuals for inherited conditions, their interests in not knowing may be relegated to second place behind the state's interest in obtaining the information. The recently-announced major government investment in genetics[24] strengthens this possibility, which undermines the previously discussed notion of 'individual' information.

---

[21] Gostin LO (1995) Genetic privacy. *Journal of Law Medical & Ethics.* **23**: 320.
[22] [1991] 71 DR 143.
[23] (1997) 45 BMLR 107.
[24] DH (2003) *Cmnd 5791.* The Stationery Office, London.

The government's agenda in the White Paper *Our Inheritance, Our Future: realising the potential of genetics in the NHS*[25] stresses the benefits to be gained from the use of genetic techniques. Its vision is 'that the NHS should lead the world in taking maximum advantage of the application of the new genetic knowledge for the benefit of all patients'.[26] To this end, the government allocated £30 million in 2002, with a pledge to invest a further £50 million in England, 'in developing genetics knowledge, skills and provision within the NHS'.[27] The potential benefits of genetics form the basis for these investments. The White Paper, for example, says that 'greater knowledge of genetics will have a major impact of our understanding of human illnesses and herald a step-change in disease prevention, diagnosis and treatment'.[28] Nonetheless, the White Paper also recognises that 'there are difficult moral issues raised by genetics advances'[29] and these issues are legal too.

Outstanding legal issues will include:

- the need to develop systems, such as those described by Gostin,[30] which are robust in protecting privacy rights
- a careful evaluation of the legitimacy (and effectiveness) of screening programmes (in respect of which the White Paper is very positive)
- consideration of the potential impact on liberties in the arena of reproduction.

Moreover, while discrimination becomes a real possibility – one which is much feared by the population – in the areas of employment and insurance, it will also become increasingly relevant in the healthcare arena. Current legal regulation of employers' behaviour will need to be strengthened and the insurance industry's voluntary codes may need to be replaced by legislative interventions designed to ensure both that privacy rights are respected and that individuals are given a fair hearing (Article 6) when disputes arise.

Globalisation

The threat posed by the easy movement of people in terms of spreading disease is also likely to create a tension between individual autonomy and more communitarian philosophies. Some developments in science, such as xenotransplantation, have a global impact which is unlike the one-to-one relationships which have characterised healthcare in the past. The major challenge for the (UK) law will lie in accommodating increased pressure for individual rights vindication and the developing global nature of health and wellbeing. The importance of international law is likely to increase with the globalisation of industries and medical research and the spread of disease between nations. Whatever the ethical debate, law is both directly and indirectly involved in regulating these areas, for example by delineating the liability of biotechnology and pharmaceutical companies, and regulating international travel. The international community is also taking an

---

[25] id.
[26] id.
[27] id.
[28] at p. 7
[29] id.
[30] Gostin LO (1995) Genetic privacy. *Journal of Law Medical & Ethics.* **23**: 320.

increasingly active interest in areas of direct relevance to health and wellbeing, for example as can be seen in the Council of Europe's Convention on Human Rights and the Convention for Protection of Human Rights and Dignity of the Human Being with Regard to the Application of Biology and Medicine: Convention on Human Rights and Biomedicine (1997).[31]

Policy recommendations

- There needs to be an explicit acknowledgement that future policy for health and healthcare should be discussed and determined in the context of ethics and the law.
- The impact of the Human Rights Act 1998 cannot be underestimated and must be robustly addressed in shaping the nature, method and quality of services in 2020.
- There will be increased focus on individual autonomy, which will influence how people see themselves as patients or consumers and how they relate to the state as provider.
- The individual's right to challenge providers' decisions has been enhanced, requiring close attention both to the *quality* of a particular decision and the *process* by which it was reached.
- There will be tensions between the increased emphasis on individual autonomy and rights on the one hand and benefits to be gained from the acquisition and use of communal information on the other.
- A practical challenge for the law will lie in accommodating increased pressure for individual rights vindication and the developing global nature of health and wellbeing.

---

[31] Council of Europe. Oviedo, 4. IV.

Chapter 3

Ethical context

Ron Zimmern, in association with Tony Hope

Ethical discourse is concerned with reasoning about what the right thing is to do in any particular situation. Ethics differs from morality insofar as it 'operates within an established framework of values that serve as a reference from which to conduct the debate about the rightness or wrongness of an action'[1] (Mason *et al.,* 2002). In theory, this construct is also relevant to law in that it provides a framework embodying the 'public conscience' (Mason *et al.,* 2002).

This chapter provides a brief assessment of ethical issues relevant to UK health policy in 2020. It aims to consider the implications of changes that are occurring and to identify changes likely to occur. It does not provide solutions to ethical dilemmas, but rather identifies areas that policymakers need to give attention in order to develop timely and appropriate responses.

Key issues are discussed under two broad themes. The first covers ethical issues specifically relating to health and health services, such as the ethics of health promotion, public health issues, euthanasia and end-of-life issues and the distinction between medical and social care. The second pertains to general issues of governance and accountability, such as the allocation of scarce resources, state versus individual responsibility and the role of public participation in health.

A definition of disease and health

Included within 'disease', 'health', 'sickness', and 'illness' are concepts that may be relevant to the state's obligations and responsibilities (Hill, 1996). A working definition of illness establishes who needs treatment, as well as who is too sick to function and is to be excused from social obligations (Parsons, 1951a,b). By contrast, specific diseases determine the priorities for medical research (Hofmann, 2001).

Health is typically understood as a social 'good' enabling the individual to function within society, and the condition defined subjectively by the individual can refer to treatment and care on the one hand, and the prevention of causes of ill health in society, the promotion of health and the absence of disease on the other (Dargie, 2000). Disease refers to a specific condition associated with illness. Illness is really a matter of how a person feels, so one can have high blood pressure but feel fine. Sickness, from a perspective of social utility, is defined as a social handicap preventing the individual from functioning fully within society.

---

[1] Such frameworks can include 'principalism' (Hope, 2004), utilitarianism or liberal individualism; *see* (Mason *et al.,* 2002).

In 1946, the World Health Organization (WHO) proposed a definition of health as 'a state of complete, physical, mental and social wellbeing and not merely the absence of disease or infirmity' (1946). It proclaimed good health to be 'a fundamental human right and a world-wide social goal' (1999).

While this definition promotes an ideal version of health, it fails to define and measure wellbeing. WHO acknowledged that a working definition of health is needed in order to establish targets for achievement in health policy and made operational its definition of health as 'the reduction in mortality, morbidity, and disability due to detectable disease or disorder, and an increase in the perceived level of health' (1999).

However, this definition still fails to capture the complexity of the social aspects of disease and notions of disease, illness and sickness are conflated. The differences between a disease and a serious condition, for example, may be interpreted in many ways.[2]

When the word 'health' is used, it is not usually specified whether it means the absence of 'disease', 'sickness' or 'illness'. The WHO definition is clearly a sociological concept reflecting the absence of 'sickness' or 'illness': a person may function exactly as required in the definition yet harbour a growing cancer or narrowed coronary arteries. Such people are 'diseased' but not 'sick' or 'ill'. The converse is the multi-symptomatic individual with no detectable signs of 'disease'. Such people are 'sick' and it is appropriate that they receive appropriate management and services, but they are not 'diseased'.

It can be tempting to think that if only the right definition of 'disease', 'illness' or 'health' were available, the moral and ethical problems of defining the responsibility of the state or what should be taken from a healthcare budget (and what, for example, from a social services budget) would be solved. This view is almost certainly false. If finding a definition of 'illness' is to determine the services that should be provided by a state healthcare system, then the ethical issues regarding state responsibilities prior to finding the definition for 'illness' will have to be raised. Conversely, finding a definition for 'illness' free from ethical considerations will result in one that is of marginal value in terms of answering difficult ethical issues.

Medical and social care

Medical and social care are currently seen as distinct concepts in policy terms. They are carried out by different people, governed by different legal frameworks and have different funding streams.

The distinction between medical and social care has been used in England to devolve the budgetary responsibility for social care away from the NHS and on to

---

[2] For instance, what in 1993 determined high and low blood pressure and how this was treated varied. In Germany, low blood pressure will be treated whereas in the UK it often will not be, and in the US it would reduce the sufferer's life insurance. Furthermore, what would be considered treatable high blood pressure in the US might be considered normal in the UK (Davey and Popay, 1993). The definitions of high and low pressure have since changed, and what is considered high blood pressure has been lowered. Effectively, this means that more people suffer from high blood pressure (CMO, 2001).

local authorities.[3] Two questions are raised when considering whether this distinction is ethically justifiable. First, whether it is possible to draw up robust criteria for such a distinction – is it possible to separate conventionally medical care activities such as the giving of injections, the care of naso-gastric tubes or of bedsores, from conventionally social activities such as bathing, toilet care, cooking or shopping? Is the distinction meaningful? Second, even if conceptually sound, is there a morally relevant difference between these two categories of care that might justify the use of separate regulatory, financial or legal regimes?

The funding of care is a politically sensitive issue. Within confined budgets, financial advantages may be gained by moving funding responsibility. In the future, more people will have a complex mixture of health and social care needs. While previously, medical care activities have required a measure of expertise, as technology becomes more accessible in the home, the distinction between health and social care will become increasingly important.

Reduction of disability, enhancement and lifestyle interventions

A similar set of questions may be asked in relation to the distinction between enhancement of individual traits and the management of impairment or disability. Is this a conceptually meaningful distinction, and can morally relevant distinctions be made between these concepts? The answer will depend in part on notions and definitions of disease or normality. Are interventions that improve the intellectual function of a child to be regarded as the reduction of disability or the enhancement of a natural trait? Does the distinction depend on the baseline level of the trait under consideration? Is the nature of the intervention – whether social (better schooling), environmental (better diet), medical (a drug) or genetic (gene therapy) – a relevant consideration? Would it be ethically wrong, for example, to give a drug, or gene therapy, to make a child perform better at school? This question will have to be faced in the near future.

Within the current policy context, the public expect the NHS to pay for 'necessary' interventions – but how is 'necessary' to be defined? Some would regard breast augmentation surgery to be 'cosmetic', a form of enhancement, and would argue that such surgery should not fall within NHS entitlement. But would this apply in rare cases where the patient is without any significant breast tissue, or has extremely asymmetrical breasts? These examples matter when defining entitlements and resource allocation within a publicly-funded health system.

Individual or public health

Traditional ethical approaches to healthcare appear to be based on two separate and sometimes contradictory principles: the clinician's prime duty towards the individual patient, and the health service's duty to the population as a whole. Should

---

[3] Divergent policies in Scotland and England (and strong popular feeling in England) suggest that this issue is still in need of more rigorous consideration.

the ultimate goal of the health service be to maximise health (and minimise illness) overall, or to reduce inequalities? This has implications for how healthcare is created and distributed. A related issue concerns the extent to which individuals may legitimately be expected to take responsibility for improving their own health status and whether individual responsibility should be based on individuals paying for their own care.

Health promotion

Current policy emphasises health promotion (Conservative Party, 2004; DH, 2004a,b; Wanless, 2004). The report *Securing Good Health for the Whole Population* (Wanless, 2004) focuses on a 'fully engaged' scenario, in which citizens strive to optimise their own health in partnership with health professionals, predicting that this will result in significant savings in the healthcare budget and improvement to health. Although this is contentious, there is no dissent from the view that the achievement of better health at an individual or population level is desirable.

The ethical issue most important to health promotion is the extent to which the state should intervene, as distinct from merely providing knowledge, to change the behaviour of individuals with regard to having healthier lifestyles. Many people engaging in unhealthy behaviour know it is unhealthy (Abel-Smith, 1994). While the state has assumed some responsibility for addressing the wider determinants of health, such as the provision of clean air and water, it is not clear where this line should be drawn. Bambra *et al.* (2003) argue that no capitalist government will support the 'full implementation of a radical equity agenda'. Indeed, the right to life (contained in Article 2 of the Council of Europe Convention on Human Rights) has been interpreted as imposing a positive obligation on states to secure the lives of their citizens, for example, by providing effective vaccination programmes. A related question is whether it has similar responsibilities in relation to individual behaviour such as smoking, eating habits and the intake of alcohol and drugs. Are there ethical distinctions to be made between health promotion interventions?

Those who believe that health is the most important of all human goals may support programmes of behavioural change in society; while libertarians may question whether it is the government's role to do more than give its citizens the knowledge to behave in a healthy manner.[4] There are two issues about the implicit value of health promotion, which are seen to run counter to those increasingly underpinning clinical medicine. The first is regarding an individual refusing treatment, even if it is life-saving. The second concerns the paternalism inherent in health promotion practice, which negates the individual's right to engage in certain practices, such as self-harming. When should individual choice be curtailed for sake of the wider community? Where this line is drawn will depend on the relative claims of libertarian values of individual autonomy, liberty and privacy, compared with the perceived needs of the wider community. In practice, current policy focus on changing individual behaviour in order to improve health outcomes is not consistent with government inaction to address some of the well-established wider

---

[4] One might argue that the government's role in health promotion is unacceptable as it seeks ways to save money and will inevitably have a short-term focus. The question arises as to how best to engage the public in health promotion.

determinants of health. The question is whether is it ethical to neglect the wider determinants of health when there is evidence that they matter.

Futility/euthanasia

Also relating to autonomy, and a focus for demands for legislative changes, are euthanasia[5] and physician-assisted suicide.[6] A number of countries, including The Netherlands, Belgium and Switzerland, have liberalised the law with regard to these issues over the last few years and undoubtedly other countries will follow suit. The pressure to liberalise the law in the UK will come from the examples in other countries, from the fact that some UK citizens will travel to countries where such options are legal (such as 'suicide tourism' to Switzerland) and from the push towards respect for patient autonomy within the domestic sphere. An inevitable corollary of extending choice of treatment is to extend the choice not to have treatment.[7]

The pressure to keep the *status quo* may come from perceived experiences abroad and the related fear of a 'slippery slope'. The House of Lords has rejected the issue of legalising euthanasia on two main grounds: that it is a practice at odds with the sanctity of life and that it is unnecessary because it is possible to control pain and other suffering through other means. The sanctity of life argument may ultimately be sustainable only within a religious framework and if the power of such a framework continues to decline,[8] this argument may decrease in political force. Lord Joffe's Assisted Dying for the Terminally Ill Bill and the House of Lords Select Committee that has been set up is an example of this (House of Lords, 2004). On the other hand, advances in medical technology may render the second of these grounds increasingly powerful. No scientific advance is likely to overcome non-pain based suffering, however, and some patients may prefer death to the side-effects of pain management.

There is evidence from Oregon, in the US, that most patients seeking assisted suicide do so from fear of losing their autonomy (Revill, 2004). Although it is clear that the Human Rights Act 1998 cannot compel states to legislate for euthanasia or physician-assisted suicide,[9] human rights jurisprudence may come to dominate the political agenda. In this context it is also worth noting that the issue of abortion has once again come under scrutiny. Arguments as to which life is to be considered an absolute priority and where life should begin and end continue to be pursued.

---

[5] In euthanasia, the patient is killed by someone other than him- or herself.

[6] In physician-assisted suicide the patient, not the physician, carries out the act of killing.

[7] A patient's advance refusal of treatment, which is a formally written document informing the doctor what kind of treatment they desire when they become incapable of making a decision, is binding on doctors under common law although it is not yet enshrined by an act of Parliament. A 'living will', which only comes into force when a patient is terminally ill and has less than six months to live, is in accord with current law as well as good medical practice, and is encouraged by the BMA and the Law Commission. The BMA currently opposes physician-assisted suicide and euthanasia, despite changes in attitude amongst doctors (Mayor, 2004), and sees 'some form of assisted death legislation inevitable' (Godfrey, 2004).

[8] Perhaps for that very reason, because religion seems to be of less significance in our lives, those who are adherents of a religious faith might be more strident in defence of their beliefs by 2020.

[9] *Pretty v United Kingdom* 66 BMLR 147, E ct HR (2002).

Resource allocation

In the future, for reasons such as demographic change, technological push and increased patient expectation and demand, the gap between the demand for healthcare and what is sought will continue to grow. Questions relating to healthcare resource distribution will remain a major issue in healthcare decision-making and will impact on the development of the overall system of healthcare delivery.

Decisions about resource allocation will continue to be made on grounds of cost-effectiveness or, more honestly, on notions of affordability, since the term 'cost-effective' is often a euphemism to disguise a rationing decision. Any decision on rationing raises ethical considerations. For example, there is a bias in clinical science where there is more excitement over rare diseases than rehabilitation.

An ethical concern is whether in the best allocation of resources for populations, the rights of individuals may be sacrificed for the greater good. A system based around cost-effectiveness would severely limit healthcare for those who are likely to have a poor prognosis even with treatment.[10] Moreover, the present methods for assessing health needs inevitably favour those with common illnesses and provide scant hope for those unfortunate enough to suffer from a rare disease. It is unclear whether the population is likely to prefer a system based mainly on consequentialist[11] regimes, informed primarily by health economic considerations, or whether it would wish the healthcare system to focus primarily on individual prognosis, to save the lives of people most likely to die.

The continuing pressure on healthcare resources will intensify the debate regarding care paid for by the individual and care covered by a socialised system. This relates to some of the issues discussed under the ethics of health promotion, and whether a socialised health system should provide care for those who have behaved 'irresponsibly' (Hill, 1996).

In addition, the push for collecting cost-effectiveness data (and the broader interest in evidence-based medicine and evidence-based population health policies) will raise the issue of whether healthcare provided through national funding should be delivered within a research framework. In such a framework, the *quid pro quo* of state provision is that patients allow data from their healthcare to be used for research purposes to increase the cost-effectiveness of future treatments and policy analysis.

The issue of how resources should be allocated to research is key to the issue of how resources should be spent in the future. Future treatment options will be dependent on current research. A related issue concerns the extent to which big business drives the research agenda – a pertinent issue in the future because policy is already moving in that direction without resolving ethical tensions.

Partnership with the private sector

Ethical questions arise concerning private partnerships in health and in scientific and medical research. Recent policy documents envisage greater collaboration

---

[10] Palliative care is overlooked by quality-adjusted life year calculations. It is also ignored for the reason that the patients are not ill but dying. *See* the Nuffield Trust Buckinghamshire Declaration on care for the dying.

[11] The doctrine that the morality of an action is to be judged solely by its consequences.

between academic and commercial sectors, with universities and the NHS being exhorted to pay greater attention to technology transfer and intellectual property (HM Treasury, 2003). Innovation and competitiveness appear high on the political agenda, but this raises questions about whether these developments may be reconciled with a nationalised system of healthcare delivery, and whether they are necessary or desirable. Will such partnerships distort the research agenda?[12] There is evidence that the general public is suspicious of the use of public finance for private enterprise (Royal Society and Royal Academy of Engineering, 2003).[13]

These considerations may give additional strength to issues relating to the commodification of body parts and of health information – issues of ownership and privacy, and what should be private and what public in health and healthcare.

On the other hand, 21st Century science requires resources from the private sector. Moreover, it is certainly true that the development of healthcare products, diagnostic and therapeutic, has always been the responsibility of the commercial sector, and that such development necessitates that shareholders are compensated for the risk that they take in investing in the development process. Another question is whether public money should be used for private enterprise and whether it should create private profit.

Research ethics and information

Current trends toward greater protection of individual 'rights' are having an effect on the cost and possibility of research.[14] Discussions of consent and ownership raise complex ethical questions: should an individual patient have complete control over the use of her data, and must that consent always be sought? Or should society seek only to ensure that such patients are not harmed, whether physically or psychologically, when such data are used? If the latter view were taken, it would be deemed ethical to use anonymised data without consent.

Genetic data, by which most people mean data derived from the analysis of DNA or other genetic material, provides another source of ethical debate. The view that it requires a separate regulatory regime, known as genetic exceptionalism, should be resisted. Personal data, including genetic data, must be adequately protected, but the arguments that genetic data require a greater degree of protection than other types of health data are not compelling. Hope (2004) illustrates the shared nature of genetic information using the example of a woman who knows she is a carrier of the Duchenne Muscular Dystrophy mutation. She holds information relevant to herself and her children, but also relevant to her sister and her children. In this example, it is clear that the information is relevant to her family, but it is relevant because of the special nature of the disease rather than the special nature of the data

---

[12] Some of these issues were explored in a special edition of the *British Medical Journal* in 2003 (BMJ, 2003), focusing on the relationship of the pharmaceutical industry with clinicians, researchers, patient groups and medical journals. However, as noted by Kmietowicz 'funding from any source, whether from government, charitable bodies, or drug companies, has strings attached' (Kmietowicz, 2004).

[13] US survey evidence also suggests that the public does not think that pharmaceutical companies generally do a good job of serving their customers (*The Economist*, 2004).

[14] The Human Tissue Act discussed in Chapter 7 provides a good example.

(Parker and Lucassen, 2004). Care must be taken not to conflate genetic information meaning 'information about DNA' and genetic information meaning 'information (however derived) about an inherited disorder'.

Healthcare management – professional autonomy and targets

Clinical staff and health service managers experience ethical tensions between addressing the needs of their patients and imposed management imperatives and performance measures. Healthcare professionals argue that primary accountability should be to the patient, while management considerations dictate that it must be to the organisation, by meeting its objectives and demands. Clinical professionals and managers face the problem that doing what is best for individual patients or for the community is often in conflict with the need to meet politically-determined targets. Trying to reduce waiting lists in one specialty, for example, can negatively impact on others irrespective of clinical need; or may mandate inappropriate treatment decisions based on meeting targets rather than clinical need. At present, there appears to be variation across the devolved territories, for example, professionals in Scotland are allowed greater autonomy than those in England (Greer, 2005).

This divergence reflects widespread agreement among health professionals that performance and audit trends have probably gone too far and that these measures, and associated regulatory regimes, distort the practice of medicine and the conduct of scientific and medical research (Academy of Medical Sciences, 2003; O'Neill, 2002; Wellcome Trust, 2004).

There are ethical implications if meeting performance targets affects ways in which resources are utilised, or results in inappropriate patient management. In order for a general practice to receive full payment for cervical smears, it will need to achieve a target level of coverage for women to undergo the procedure. This puts pressure on the doctors to persuade women to have a cervical smear rather than simply to inform them about the procedure. It may be argued that meeting a performance target requires the use of coercion and may not meet the requirements of fully-informed consent. Against this, it may be argued that high coverage is necessary to ensure that the greatest number of incipient cancers are detected and dealt with to the benefit of the individual women. While informed choice is currently being debated in screening circles, the costs and the benefits of using performance targets in healthcare – and the philosophical basis of concepts such as consent, privacy and confidentiality – are matters requiring detailed critical scrutiny.

Lay and public power – choice and participation

Current policies focusing on choice and 'putting people at the heart of public services' (DH, 2004c) suggest that in the future, particularly in England, greater lay or public involvement is likely (Greer, 2004). While this may prove more responsive to public demands, it could also lead to inappropriate provision of services and be to the detriment of the most effective provision. Gostin (2004) and Hope (2001;

2004) have noted how the 'rescue imperative' – the process by which resources are allocated to futile endeavours just to prevent death or for the benefit of seriously ill individuals for whom the probability of cure or improvement is low – can distort decisions regarding allocation. It is not that one position is 'right or wrong', but rather that the issue is an open one requiring consideration.

Furthermore, satisfaction of patient demand is not the only outcome important to healthcare. Matters of equity and justice must also be considered, as must the sources of patient demand. It is important to be aware that demand is often generated as a result of commercial rather than patient interests. There are important legal questions about the extent to which existing consumer legislation and regulations protect the public and ensure that only efficacious remedies are allowed in the marketplace. This raises conceptions of efficacy, and of who in society should define it. A libertarian approach may take the view that the role of the state should go no further than to regulate access to products that are unsafe, and that those that are safe but ineffective are the concern of the consumer for whom the maxim *caveat emptor* should suffice.

In terms of public engagement, there is no single public interest. The interests of some people (such as those at risk of a particular disease) may conflict with the interests of others in terms of resource allocation and health promotion interventions. There may also be a danger that powerful minorities and specific interest groups will dominate, leading to injustice. This does not render the principle of patient power unethical, but raises the question of how patient wishes and views can properly affect healthcare decisions whilst not leading to injustice – how democracy and rational ethical deliberation are balanced. Some will argue for a greater role for patients and the public on ethical grounds because participation in itself supports autonomy and personal responsibility (Halpern *et al.,* 2004).

Globalisation

Growing trends in globalisation – such as the increasing ability of people to move from country to country in order to access healthcare, access to information from across the world via the Internet, international guidelines and the growing importance of European law – raise several ethical issues relevant to future UK health policy. First, each country has to consider what should be illegal, in the knowledge that some people will be able to access healthcare that is illegal in their own country by travelling abroad.[15] Should this affect the laws that are enacted?

Second, it is increasingly possible for individuals to find out and compare healthcare in other countries. This will lead to pressure on each healthcare system to provide care comparable with the best elsewhere. International guidelines are becoming increasingly important, and even when not formally part of law, they can exert considerable authority. This has been particularly relevant in the regulation of medical research. European law is beginning to affect practice in the UK and this effect is likely to increase.

---

[15] *R v Human Fertilisation and Embryology Authority, ex p Blood* (Hope) 2 All ER 687.

To some extent, globalisation results in less freedom for a country to solve ethical (and practical) problems in isolation. It also poses the problem of what to do when there is a conflict between 'international' pressure (such as an international guideline) and what most people in the country think is right. This in turn puts pressure on healthcare resources as patients make demands based on comparisons with other countries, although some pressures could lead to increased funding for healthcare.

The globalisation of businesses means that large multinational companies are likely to have increasing power within individual countries. This power may be used in the interests of company owners rather than in the interests of the population of each country.

Policy process

There are often no right answers to difficult ethical questions, particularly when ethical principles conflict with real life situations. Proper processes ensure a degree of legitimacy for the decisions that are taken. Explicit processes and principles have been developed by health authorities and primary care trusts, for example, as to how they prioritise resource allocation decisions. The courts will examine these closely in deciding the legitimacy of a decision if challenged at judicial review.

Is proper process sufficient in itself? Is it also necessary to bear in mind the quality of the decision and the arguments used? How is critical reflection by a properly-constituted group of individuals (such as the Human Fertilisation and Embryology Authority or the Human Genetics Commission) to be reconciled with basic tenets of democracy, when public opinion is for one view whereas critical reflection leads to another? Can and should public consultation and engagement ever determine the 'ought' of an ethical question?

Policy recommendations

- There needs to be an explicit acknowledgement that future policy for health and healthcare should be discussed and determined in the context of ethics and the law.
- There are currently tensions between increased emphasis on individual autonomy and rights, and a paternalism inherent in health promotion and more communitarian responses necessary for addressing globalisation.
- Ethical and legal positions change with generations, technological developments and dominant ideology, as well as with wider attitudinal changes in society. In an increasingly secular society, for example, sanctity of life might cease to be a justification for not changing the law on euthanasia.
- One major policy challenge will be to find ways to support sufficient convergence of interests and views of individual citizens, patients and carers, representatives of communities and populations, individual and peer groups of clinical professionals, research scientists and technology developers and agents of the state.
- Another policy challenge will be addressing the tension between what is best for a population as a whole and individual choices and rights.

- Thought needs to be given to the *process* by which ethical issues are addressed. By which process might a distinction between disability and enhancement be drawn, or health defined as an individual or public good? Consideration also needs to be given to implications for responsibility and payment.

References

Abel-Smith B (1994) Lifestyle and health promotion. In: *An introduction to Health: policy, planning, and financing.* Longman Publishing, New York, pp. 33–45.

Academy of Medical Sciences (2003) *Strengthening Clinical Research.* The Academy of Medical Sciences, London.

Bambra C, Fox D and Scott-Samuel A (2003) *Toward a New Politics of Health.* Politics of Health Group, University of Liverpool, Liverpool.

BMJ (2003) Pharma industry. *British Medical Journal.* **326.**

CMO (2001) *On the State of the Public Health.* Department of Health, London.

Conservative Party (2004) *Right to Choose. Health Issue.* The Conservative Party, London.

Dargie C (2000) *Policy Futures for UK Health. 2000 Report.* The Nuffield Trust, London.

Davey B and Popay J (1993) *Dilemmas in Health Care.* Open University Press, Buckingham.

DH (2004a) All NHS doctors by country of primary medical qualification. Personal Communication. Email to: Chang LR.

DH (2004b) *Choosing Health: making healthier choices easier. Cmnd 6374.* Department of Health, London.

DH (2004c) *The NHS Improvement Plan: putting people at the heart of public services.* Department of Health, London.

Godfrey K (2004) BMA continues to oppose assisted suicide and euthanasia. *British Medical Journal.* **329:** 997.

Gostin LO (2004) *Health of the People: the highest law.* Queen Elizabeth II Conference Centre, London.

Greer S (2004) *Four Way Bet: how devolution has led to four different models for the NHS.* University College London, London.

Greer S (2005) Why do good politics make bad health policy? In: S Dawson and C Sausman (eds) *Future Health Organisations and Systems.* Palgrave Macmillan, Basingstoke.

Halpern D, Bates C, Beales G and Heathfield A (2004) *Personal Responsibility and Changing Behaviour: the state of knowledge and its implications for public policy.* Prime Minister's Strategy Unit, London.

Hill TP (1996) Health care: a social contract in transition. *Social Science & Medicine.* **43**(5): 783–9.

HM Treasury (2003) *Lambert Review of Business–University Collaboration. Final Report.* HM Treasury, London.

Hofmann B (2001) Complexity of the concept of disease as shown through rival theoretical frameworks. *Theoretical Medicine and Bioethics.* **22**(3): 211–36.

Hope T (2001) Rationing and life-saving treatment: should identifiable patients have higher priority? *Journal of Medical Ethics.* **27**(3):179–85.

Hope T (2004) *Medical Ethics: a very short introduction.* Oxford University Press, Oxford.

House of Lords (2004) *Assisted Dying for the Terminally Ill Bill.* TSO, London.

Kmietowicz Z (2004) Tighter controls are needed to root out bogus patient groups. *British Medical Journal.* **329:** 1307.

Mason JK, McCall Smith RA and Laurie GT (2002) *Law and Medical Ethics.* Butterworths, London.

Mayor S (2004) UK body calls on UN to allow for therapeutic cloning. *British Medical Journal*. **329**: 938.

O'Neill O (2002) Reith Lectures 2002: A question of trust. http://www.bbc.co.uk/radio4/reith2002/lecture4.shtml. Accessed: 3 October 2004.

Parker M and Lucassen A (2004) Genetic information: a joint account? *British Medical Journal*. **329**: 165–7.

Parsons T (1951a) Illness and the role of the physician: a sociological perspective. *American Journal of Orthopsychiatry*. **21**: 452–60.

Parsons T (1951b) *The Social System*. Free Press, Chicago.

Revill J (2004) Death on doctor's orders. http://society.guardian.co.uk/print/0,3858,5078724–105965,00.html. Accessed: 6 December 2004.

Royal Society and Royal Academy of Engineering (2003) *Nanotechnology: views of scientists and engineers*. The Royal Society and Royal Academy of Engineering, London.

The Economist (2004) *Got a match?* http://www.economist.com/displaystory.cfm?story_id=3432570. Accessed: 31 March 2005.

Wanless D (2004) *Securing Good Health for the Whole Population. Final Report*. HM Treasury, London.

Wellcome Trust (2004) *Public Health Sciences: challenges and opportunities. Report of the Public Health Sciences Working Group convened by the Wellcome Trust*. The Wellcome Trust, London.

WHO (1946) *Preamble to the Constitution of the World Health Organization as adopted by the International Health Conference, New York, 19–22 June*. World Health Organization, Geneva.

WHO (1999) *Health 21: health for all in the 21st century*. World Health Organization Regional Office for Europe, Copenhagen.

Part 2

Analysing key policy issues

Chapter 4

Who's going to govern?[1]

Zoë Slote Morris and Sandra Dawson

A factor central to the future of UK health policy is the role the state will play in terms of healthcare provision and the promotion of improving health status for the population. In the UK, the state still provides 80% of healthcare, funded through taxation and free to all at the point of delivery. The commitment to 'socialised medicine' and to the belief that health is fundamentally 'a public good' creates a special relationship between the state and society (Dawson and Sausman, 2005). This in turn creates a special relationship between the electorate, politicians, civil servants, those involved in the NHS as patients, carers, clinicians and executives, and those involved from various sectors in areas which affect health status but which are not part of the NHS (Mulligan and Appleby, 2001).

This chapter considers the role of the state and issues of governance in future UK health policy. Health policy in the UK continues to be highly centralised in terms of planning and provision, at macro and micro levels, despite some devolution to the home countries. So why is the state involved in healthcare? There are two reasons. The first is that healthcare in the UK is mainly funded through taxation, and the second is that health is conceived as a public good. The state is therefore held responsible for meeting certain expectations. These include delivering value for money, ensuring high quality and preventing what is perceived as avoidable ill health and disease. A major challenge for public policy is that of ever-rising expectations fuelled by scientifically-revealed possibilities (*see* Chapter 7), international comparisons and a sense of what is 'right' and what are 'individual rights' (*see* Chapters 2 and 3, and the section on 'Information, evaluation and benchmarking' in Chapter 9).

Issues emerging from a wider consideration of the state in UK health have been selected because of their potential impact on UK health (including public health) or because of their current status in health policy (such as patient choice). Dawson and Sausman (2005) suggest a framework for analysis which includes a focus on the scope of the system (state responsibilities, citizens' entitlements); ownership of the

---

[1] The authors use the word 'govern' to refer to the 'conduct of policy and affairs of [a state, organisation or people]'. In this context, it is a state, describing a political-geographical entity: 'a nation or territory considered as an organised political community under one government' (OUP, 1999). Dunleavy and O'Leary (1987) identify two sorts of definitions of the state: organisational and functional. Functional definitions may be *ex ante* – 'a set of institutions which carries out particular goals, purposes and objectives' – or *ex post*, in which case the state is defined by its consequences. Organisational definitions tend to conceive the state as 'a set of governmental institutions ... synonymous with the elected ministers who are formally in charge in the departments' (Dunleavy and O'Leary, 1987); often used interchangeably with government, and meaning the Executive.

system (funding, organisation and accountability); stakeholders (including patients, society and the workforce) and 'dynamics' (a term used to describe the mechanisms that drive the system). Each of these is relevant to the role of the state because it is the state that specifies entitlements, funding arrangements and dynamics.

The role of the state in health policy

In considering the overall policy canvas for state involvement, it is important to bear in mind that a range of involvement across a range of arenas is possible (Rice, 1995). Typically, policy and analysis tend to focus on the National Health Service (NHS) as an institution and the use of public money in health. Yet many factors relating to health, such as developments in technology, or the physical and social environment, lie in other arenas. Regarding the governance of future health policy, the state has a far greater impact owing to its activities across other arenas, and far greater scope for intervention than is often perceived to be the case.

Coupled with this is the notion of who does what within the health system. Klein (2005), for example, has identified a move away from the identification of one institution in the provision of health services, namely the NHS. This is reflected in greater and more explicit use of private providers and the 'third sector'. At the same time, within a single policy area there are ranges of functions which a state may assume and the resulting landscape of state provision, regulation and *laissez faire* is influenced by historical, economic and ideological considerations. One important area for future consideration in the UK is the relation of social care to health and healthcare. While ministerial responsibility for both is combined, the role of government with regard to each differs. For social care, government is perceived as determining the underlying policy values and regulating activities but taking an 'arm's length' role in relation to funding and direct provision through means-tested access to public provision. On the other hand, with regard to most of what is called 'health' care, the role of government has been to determine the underlying policy values, to regulate activities and directly to fund and provide services free of charge at the point of access. This creates an immediate source of political and public confusion and will need to be addressed in the future.

This chapter focuses on what is considered to be of most relevance to the present and future health policy agenda of the UK: the role of the state in relation to other governance authorities, to markets, and to the professions and individuals. In doing so, it is worth remembering that the involvement of any state could be either much more or much less, it could even have a different role, depending on historical, economic and social factors.

This chapter focuses on scope and stakeholders through an examination of the state's relationships with other actors in the policy system. There are four main sections:

- the state as embodied in central government and its relationship to supranational, UK home country and local government
- the state and the market
- the state and the health professions – particularly in relation to regulation and performance management

- the state and the citizen – with particular emphasis on the role of the patient and public in health.

Themes and examples are designed to be illustrative and are not exhaustive.

The state and other governance authorities

A key driver of the shift towards governance is the devolution and potential 'hollowing-out' of the state (Rhodes, 1996). Hollowing-out involves passing responsibility upwards to supranational bodies, such as the European Union (EU), and downwards to devolved countries, or further, to regions. It suggests that nation states will become increasingly redundant in the future. The likely impacts of this on future UK health policy are considered in turn.

The European Union

European law takes precedence over national law. Three tenets of European law with direct implications for health are:

- free movement of goods, e.g. medical technology, pharmaceuticals
- persons, e.g. patients, health professionals
- services, e.g. health services.

In two landmark cases in July 2000, the European Court of Justice (ECJ) ruled that patients were entitled to seek treatment in another member state without prior authorisation by their national health service, unless treatment could be provided domestically without 'undue delay' (BMA, 2003).

European legislation is impacting on healthcare services in other ways, with the implementation of the European Social Chapter and the Working Time Directive limiting the hours medical staff are permitted to work. Implications for NHS staffing are significant as organisations such as hospitals strive to increase medical staff numbers and redesign staffing models. The impact of the European Convention on Human Rights, enshrined in the UK Human Rights Act, is also anticipated to have a profound effect on health and healthcare in the UK in future (*see* Chapters 2 and 5). Article 152 of the Amsterdam Treaty (1997) specifically extended public health governance to the EU.

Since its inception under the Treaty of Rome in 1957, the EU has left direct competency for healthcare to its member states. Subsequent treaties, such as the Single European Act (1987), the Maastricht Treaty (1992) and the Amsterdam Treaties (1997), failed to enlarge EU competence in health beyond aspects of public health, including health service provision and health system financing. Few direct powers have so far been ceded, although the impact of the EU may be felt more indirectly in future. What is emerging is somewhat complicated. The proposed constitution is explicit about not extending EU competence to healthcare. At the same time the four freedoms of the EU – freedom of movement of goods, services, capital and people – are all being enforced by the European Court of Justice with ramifications for health services. For example, freedom of movement has been interpreted as freedom to use health services in another country while billing the NHS, and freedom of services means countries cannot discriminate against professionals from anywhere else in the EU. The Services Directive reinforces this trend, resulting in some concerns that the EU will, in time, regulate many aspects of UK healthcare policy (Greer, 2005). However, the Services Directive was revised in May 2005. The likely impact of this is still unclear.

The home countries

With regard to devolution to the home countries within the UK, 'the extent of policy divergence since devolution has surprised many' (Greer, 2004). This makes any discussion of UK policy as a whole somewhat problematic. Although health policy within each of the four countries is framed within the same statutory framework and they each face similar broad future challenges (BMA, 2004), the differences between them are substantive (BBC, 2004a,b,c,d). The countries diverge over how to meet goals but there are few signs of learning going 'upwards' in terms of sharing of best practice or policy solutions from one country to another. One advantage of this divergence is that it provides a natural experiment. If governments are committed to improving health policy based on evidence, one of their roles might be to better understand and evaluate divergence. Leatherman and Sutherland's (2005) study of quality in the NHS does find differences between countries.

Localising policy

Another aspect of devolution central to the provision of healthcare is the move to empower frontline staff, with an increased policy focus on 'responsive' public services. Thus, *Shifting the Balance of Power: the next steps* (DH, 2002) aimed to move from a top-down approach, emphasising national standards and accountability, towards local leadership and accountability. Few would argue that this agenda has been successfully pursued (Baggott, 2004). Indeed, *Shifting the Balance of Power* was itself published against a backdrop of greater central control – in the form of the establishment of the Modernisation Agency, CHAI, NICE and National Service Frameworks (NSFs), for example – as well as increasing centralisation of funds attached to central initiatives (Baggott, 2004). Focus is on central targets with regular and intrusive monitoring (Day and Klein, 1987 cited in Walshe, 2002) and local commissioners continue to commission within a centrally-defined framework.

This has led to some discussion of the need to redesign the health service to allow greater freedom from government. The Commission on the NHS has suggested that the NHS be established as a public corporation with a constitution protecting its founding principles, its own board and operating freedoms (Hutton, 2000). A King's Fund report (2002) also argued for the separation of government and health service through the establishment of an NHS corporation. Government would establish policy objectives and allocate resources, but the NHS corporation would decide how to meet these objectives and assume responsibility for standards and regulation, as well as local resource allocation (*see also* Dewar, 2003).

There are, however, issues of jurisdiction and responsibility. Politicians may think that they would not and should not relinquish control, since most healthcare in the UK is funded through public money. Baggott (2004) argues that separate agency status will not resolve the issues of ministers needing to take responsibility. The desire to empower the frontline and maintain accountability and control is an old dilemma on which there has been little progress towards a resolution.

According to Smee (1995):

*Ministers and the centre are finding it difficult to reconcile devolved account-
ability with the demand for detailed monitoring created by parliamentary interest
in operational issues. In consequence, the centre is drawn into a whole range of
issues, from hospital catering standards to freedom of speech for hospital staff,
that it once expected to leave to the discretion of local management. The dilemma
is that without substantial operating freedom, trust management cannot be expected
to produce better performance ... but that with such freedom there is bound to be
diversity of behaviours and performance. The existence of outliers is there to be
seen – by press, auditors and politicians – as a cause for central regulation.*

Complicating matters further is the fact there is more to health than healthcare,
although the relinquishing of direct control over the healthcare system does not
necessarily imply a retreat of government from other arenas relevant to health.
Some (for example Dewar, 2003) argue that new arrangements would result in
greater democratic deficit and that such reforms are impossible anyway because
universal health has to be centralised and hierarchical to achieve the wider goals.
Bambra *et al.* (2003) point out health is an inescapably political activity and should
not be taken out of the political arena.

The wider determinants of health are amenable to political action: health is not
equally distributed and improving health requires collective activity at the societal
level – 'health can only be improved through the organised activities of communities and societies. The organisation of society, in most countries, is the role of the
state and its agencies' (Bambra *et al.*, 2003). Health is perceived to be a social right
(Marshall, 1963) and is therefore relevant to citizenship. Increasingly too, health
assumes a political relevance in the context of increasing globalisation.

Important issues need to be addressed regarding the central-local balance.
Should the 'outliers' to which Smee (1995) referred, for example, be viewed as a
social menace or benign inevitabilities? Will communities prefer local responsiveness or national standards? What if local choices impact on population health?
Localisation may also imply a greater role of local or regional government, or a shift
in ownership of the healthcare infrastructure (Bosanquet *et al.*, 2003). Will this
negate the idea of a 'national' service, and will it matter?

If these basic questions can be answered, then the policy issue becomes one of
designing appropriate structures and instruments. There may be scope to learn from
examples in Wales, where a more localist agenda has been pursued (Greer, 2004). It
is clear, however, that for the most part attempts to shift the balance within current
healthcare arrangements have hitherto been unsuccessful, instead resulting in
more centralisation of purpose and control. Walshe (2002) suggests that NHS
regulation looks like a strengthening of central control over managerial and clinical
practice. Various regulatory bodies are set up and funded by the Department of
Health and then charged with enforcing national regulations, thereby eliminating
scope for local variation. Walshe (2002) argues that this is not inevitable if
politicians can be persuaded to 'let go'.

The state and the market

Many post-1979 UK government policies reflect an ideological preference for markets over state bureaucracies. In UK health policy, three major shifts have occurred in terms of state–market relationships. The first is greater use of the private sector to deliver services. The second shift is the attempt to mimic markets within the health system itself, following the arguments put forward by the American economist, Enthoven (1985).[2] This is reflected in a purchaser–supplier divide and greater use of contracts, for instance. These are best described as 'quasi-markets' since the purchasing powers are not with the individual. The third shift is the state's abandonment of direct provision of some services, for example dentistry, optician services and many ancillary services.[3] Thus, players in UK health markets include suppliers, intermediaries and recipients/buyers – in and between the 'internal', commercial and third sector markets – and representatives and individuals in civil society.

Healthcare services have not shifted wholesale to the private sector, but current policy, in England at least, looks certain to make more use of the private firms. A recent *Guardian* article suggests that PCTs have been instructed to include one private provider among the choices offered to patients (Dean, 2004). In a recent review of health policy in England, the former health policy advisor to the Prime Minister, Simon Stevens, explained how government is stimulating a mixed economy, or 'plurality', 'to expand capacity, enhance contestability and offer choice' (2004). Both major political parties support greater use of private providers in healthcare (Conservative Party, 2005; Reid, 2005).

The following section identifies some of the contested issues about the use of markets in UK healthcare:

- democratic deficit in accountability for policy and practice
- the principle of public money being used to fund private firms
- the impact of markets on values and the precedence afforded to 'market' values over more 'social' values – efficiency, choice and quality rather than equity and planning and the ability of markets in health to support choice.

While greater 'plurality' charts the apparent direction of public policy, there is a continuing debate about the ideological bases and practical consequences of policies and practices that create an ever-uncertain policy context.

Democratic deficit

The blurring of the line between public and private, and the fragmentation of the state, impacts on democratic control and accountability (Rhodes, 1996). It increases central government's proclivity to regulate and audit, and runs counter to current policy attempts to re-engage citizens and rejuvenate democracy. This in turn may

---

[2] Enthoven's (1985) efficiency and responsiveness argument rested on rewarding the most efficient providers, which did not happen in practice in any systematic sense in the 1990s reforms. It remains to be seen what happens with payment by results.
[3] The NHS still provides some dentistry and more complicated optician services.

contribute to declining social capital, which has direct implications for health (Harper, 2002; Lynch *et al.*, 2000; Rothstein, 2004).

Public money for private enterprise

Whether the expansion of private provision of public services can legitimately create surplus value for private appropriation is questionable. Following on from this, is use of the private sector distorting relationships and diverting policy? A recent MORI poll found that a large minority (38%) of respondents believed that 'private companies should not be involved in providing public services under any circumstances' (MORI, 2004). At the same time, a study by the National Consumer Council, suggests that service users do not care who provides the service, as long as it is good (NCC, 2004).

The role of private provision in supporting the overall aims of UK healthcare is not clear either. Pollock *et al.* (2002) argue that Private Finance Initiative (PFI) hospitals are planned on the basis of financial, as opposed to clinical, need and by means of an expensive process. Ultimately, their argument proceeds, the PFI hospitals reduce staff numbers 'in direct contradiction to government policy' and offer fewer public beds than are needed. Nonetheless, there is considerable press coverage on the role of Treatment Centres in reducing costs within the system overall (Hawkes, 2004; Kavanaugh, 2004; Timmins, 2004).

Private sector treatment is, however, often more expensive (Hawkes, 2004), not necessarily of better quality (Higgins and Wiles, 1992) and not always able to perform the difficult and expensive procedures (Baggott, 1998). Typically, the private sector has provided care in areas that are more straightforward and profitable (Baggott, 1998). Some expect this to continue as Treatment Centres spread. The Centres will choose to treat people whose condition is not complex and difficult, while expensive cases will be treated in the NHS, undermining the value of equity, which is said to underpin the health service.[4]

While considering the role of the private sector in any major segment of society, government will be aware of its role in industrial development and economic prosperity. The life sciences industry embraces pharmaceuticals, medical devices and a whole range of facilities, services and goods, in addition to private sector health and social care suppliers. Beyond its direct activities, the state has relevance to higher education as an employer of highly-skilled workers and as a sponsor of research. For all these reasons the relation of the state to the health market extends beyond this discussion and forms an important part of the policy context for UK health.

Future policy anticipates a much closer relationship between the public (government and the NHS) and private industry in health technology development (Department of Trade and Industry, 2003; HM Treasury, 2003). Governments may have to convince the private sector that it is worthwhile for them to innovate within the cost-constraints of the NHS, while persuading a cynical public that such links are positive ones. A recent article in *The Economist* noted how the pharmaceutical

---

[4] Incidentally, the same concerns are expressed within the NHS PCTs and Hospital Trusts in the context of payment by results and patient choice, where poor outcomes resulting from treatment of high-risk patients will result in patients with choice choosing to go elsewhere (Mythen and Coffey, 2004).

industry was taking public relations advice from the tobacco industry (*The Economist*, 2004).

Market versus social values

The use of commercial organisations may also result in a displacement of values. If future governments wish to remain committed to the core principles of the NHS as currently stated (Wanless, 2001), this mismatch should be addressed.

There are three areas of concern regarding values relevant to the state and future health policy. First, policymakers face choices between 'conflicting goods' in some regards (Maynard, 2005), and should understand why certain values are privileged over others (Williams, 2005). Second, even if values are explicit they are not always coherent (Greener, 2004). Third, current espoused values underpinning policy are not always reflected in practice. For example, increasing empowerment of the individual patient sits alongside a broadening and deepening of compulsion in the proposed Mental Health Bill in England.[5]

The value of choice is attracting particular attention. The private sector is seen to be central to this for increasing capacity overall and supporting more individualised care. A number of complex issues regarding values, however, are bound to arise. There is confusion about the meaning of 'consumerism' in health. Public services, of which health and social care are part, exist to fill 'market failures', and many entanglements with them are enforced differently to other services (for example, those subject to treatment under the Mental Health Act), or take place when things go wrong (Clarke, 2004). The corollary is that public services may not all be amenable to marketisation and a consumer orientation. Greener found, for instance, that people were 'bewildered' by the idea of choosing a GP and relied on their GP to select appropriate treatment for them precisely because of his or her expertise (Greener, 2003).

For markets to bring about choice and efficiency, patients need good information and the absence of dependency on particular providers. In practice, these conditions are not often met: information is often poor and/or poorly used;[6] patients have limited 'voice' and still more limited 'exit' options; and there are power asymmetries in patient–professional relationships. Greener (2003) argues that continuous 'reform' makes markets less calculable. Healthcare users' current priorities appear to relate to quality more than choice.

---

[5] Comparing new and proposed mental health legislation in England and Scotland provides a neat example of several of these tensions, as the Scottish Act has accepted a lack of evidence and is based explicitly around values (Rushmer and Hallam, 2004).

[6] Findings from the US show that purchasers and consumers of healthcare, in general, do not use performance data in making choices (Page, 2004; Schneider and Epstein, 1998). The first explanation is that people simply do not have time to 'shop around' between needing help and accessing it (Hibbard *et al.* 1996). Other issues include comprehension problems (Vaiana and McGlynn, 2002), particularly with technical data (Robinson and Brodie, 1997); a generalised lack of trust in official data (Bentley and Nash, 1998), together with a tendency to prefer informal information (Mennemeyer *et al.*, 1997); fatalism (Hibbard and Jewett, 1997); and a lack of motivation to compare organisations due to the logistical constraints of lack of alternatives or distance from home (Schneider and Epstein, 1998). All these factors have serious implications for the success of the current choice agenda.

If erstwhile patients become consumers, the dynamic between citizen and state is potentially altered. This may be counter-productive in the context of limited resources and concerns about declining social cohesion.[7] Clarke (2004) argues that the 'consumer' represents an individualist, privatised relationship 'mediated by the anonymity and autonomy granted by the cash-nexus'. By contrast, the 'citizen' embodies a 'collectivist conception of rights or entitlements, solidaristic relationships mediated by political agencies and public institutions'. Neither is inherently right or wrong, but each forms part of a different political project and has different implications.

There is also a debate as to whether consumerism is possible (when considering system capacity) or even desirable to individuals (Greener, 2003); whether consumers are able to make 'appropriate' or 'reasonable' choices (Clarke, 2004); and whether the current concept of choice is so narrowly defined (DH, 2004b) that it will have little significant impact (Appleby and Dixon, 2004). Furthermore, health services are still provided within a rationing culture (Office of Public Services Reform, 2002).

The state and the clinical professions

The state remains the largest trainer and employer of health professionals in the UK. A detailed consideration of the care workforce is given in Chapter 5, while this chapter focuses on whether and how the state should intervene in the practice and governance of healthcare. The state's relationship with health professionals is changing with the continued growth of performance management in the NHS. This is characterised by new regulatory mechanisms and explicit target-driven frameworks, which aim to ensure adequate levels of quality and performance and to hold individual organisations accountable within the NHS.

From the mid-1970s, there has been a diminution in medical dominance and autonomy within the NHS (and more generally). Greer (2004) would argue that this trend is less in evidence in Scotland, where doctors have maintained their status more successfully. Doctors have grown accustomed to practising within the 'biomedical model'[8] according to self-regulatory codes agreed by peers (Harrison and Ahmed, 2000). The powerful position they hold is derived from their control over diagnosis and treatment, evaluation of care, the nature and volume of medical tasks and their contractual independence. Expanded roles for management in the NHS, NICE guidance, the Health Commission and NSFs all reflect a changing

---

[7] Clarke gives a neat example of the privatisation of water, after which 'consumers' did not view it as their responsibility to use water 'responsibly' during a shortage, but blamed shortages on supply.

[8] The biomedical model is characterised by 'mind-body dualism' (assuming that the mind and body can be treated separately); a 'mechanical metaphor' in which a body is repaired like a machine; the 'technological imperative' which privileges technological interventions; reductionism, in that it focuses on the individual body as presented without considering wider social or psychological factors; and rests on the 'doctrine of specific aetiology', which describes the assumption that every disease is caused by a specific, identifiable entity (Nettleton, 1995). This has been challenged in terms of efficacy (McKeown, 1979), context (Engel, 1981), disease as a social construction (White, 1991) and 'professional medical dominance' as a socio-political project (Nettleton, 1995).

relationship between the state and the profession, as well as the patient and public (Ham and Alberti, 2002). The medical profession has also agreed to new (nego-tiated) contracts of employment, oversight by the Council of Regulation of Health-care Professions, statutory re-licensing every five years and a National Clinical Assessment Authority to assess doctors' performance (Stevens, 2004). Ham and Alberti (2002) suggest that this entire movement towards performance assessment and greater public accountability has caused significant shifts in governance between all players within the healthcare system.

Clinical governance

Clinical governance can be described as the 'system through which NHS organ-isations are accountable for continuously improving the quality of their services and safeguarding high standards of care by creating an environment in which excel-lence in clinical care will flourish' (Scally and Donaldson, 1998). It links standards of care with organisational performance, and has promoted cultural change within NHS hospitals. In 1999 Chief Executives in the NHS became responsible for clinical standards in their organisations with the Duty of Quality set out in the Health Act of 1999, and individual clinicians became accountable to them for delivering quality care. Clinical governance reflects a fundamental change in powers and responsi-bility of managers and individual clinicians. Consultants are no longer autonomous individuals but have a mutual responsibility to patients with a trust. Views on the impact of clinical governance are mixed. Donaldson (Donaldson and Gerard, 1989) argues a positive effect. Degeling *et al.* (2003) suggest that current arrangements for clinical governance could be improved, for example by re-establishing 'responsible autonomy' for clinicians. Whatever the specific mechanisms, clinical governance seems likely to remain an important part of policy in future, and with it regulation and audit, as a means of holding both clinicians and managers to account for the quality of care.

Regulation and audit

For future UK health policy there are two important questions: should the state intervene in the practice of medicine and, if so, how should it do so? On the one hand, the role of the state in ensuring efficient use of public money or better quality provision seems legitimate. Although measuring quality proves notoriously diffi-cult (Klein, 2005), a recent study by Leatherman and Sutherland (2003) concluded that quality in the NHS was, on balance, improving. Their subsequent study (2005) remains positive overall, whilst identifying some 'areas of concern', suggesting that monitoring can contribute to improvement. Evidence of improved productivity is less clear (ONS, 2004a).

On the other hand, Clarke and Newman (1997) suggest that trends for greater state regulation of clinical activity have a negative impact on public services: organisations focus inward, reducing their capacity to deal with complexity and uncertainty, and rendering working across boundaries more difficult. There is recent evidence, for example, that NHS hospital trusts have been forced to spend considerably more than normal to purchase extra capacity from the private sector in order to meet end-of-year targets (Donelly, 2004).

It can also be argued that increased intervention by the state has undermined professional autonomy (Ham and Alberti, 2002). In so doing, some argue that it has dissipated resources and made it more difficult for the professions to get on with their work (Maynard, 2005). Power (1994; 1997) refers to an audit explosion, and Walshe (2002) discusses 'inspectoral overload'. Regulation can be expensive. Walshe (2002) notes that, 'The costs of regulating the public sector in the United Kingdom in 1995 was estimated to be ... 0.3 per cent of public expenditure'. There are additional potential costs in terms of goodwill on the part of those being regulated and diversion of purpose, for example through the dysfunctional effect of performance management. Chapter 3 notes how target setting and regulation can create a tension for those working in the system between reconciling the interests of the patients and the demands of the system (*see also* Chapter 9).

If the state takes responsibility for protecting and promoting health, it has to find appropriate ways of doing so. If it is accepted that government has a role in regulation, the challenge for the future involves getting the structures and processes right. While the need to prevent overload and to ensure better coordination between different regulatory bodies has been recognised, the issue of perverse incentives needs careful consideration in the context of target setting. There may also be issues regarding developing goodwill amongst staff. Winstanley *et al.* (1995) note that shifting responsibilities requires ensuring that stakeholders are equipped for their new role. This is still a concern in the context of PCTs and their commissioning capacity.

The state and the public

There is increasing acceptance (at least on the part of governments) that the state cannot improve the population's health without greater engagement and participation from citizens. This leads to notions of 'co-production' (Halpern and Cockayne, 2004) and the 'fully engaged' patient with 'rights and responsibilities' (Wanless, 2002).

Pierre and Peters (2000) identify what they term a 'fundamental paradox'. The public expects government to have control over governing while at the same time resisting that control, either in terms of overt resistance, or by the way in which citizens interpret their role in policy-making and participation. Pierre and Peters (2000) argue that this may not mean that the government is becoming less powerful, but instead that state and society are more tightly bound through the process of governance because of the decline of deference, for example, increasing complexity. Indeed, they suggest that states might actually be strengthened through this process: whilst ceding some power in policy formulation they gain more control over implementation having 'co-opted social interests that might otherwise oppose its actions' (Pierre and Peters, 2000).

This section explores two discernable trends in the relationship between the state and the individual: public and patient involvement in health policy, and the individual and state in public health. Again, such issues in the UK context are tightly bound to the close identification of health policy with the publicly-funded NHS.

Public and patient involvement in health policy

Some attempts have been made in England to improve public input into healthcare services. These include Patient Forums,[9] patient representation on NHS boards and the election of boards for Foundation Hospitals. Whether these will prove effective remains to be seen (Newman, 2001), though there is little evidence to suggest much public interest in this sort of engagement.[10] Twenty per cent of locally-elected governors seats for foundation hospitals, for example, were uncontested (HSJ, 2004).

Florin and Dixon (2004) define public involvement as 'the involvement of members of the public in strategic decisions about health services and policy at local or national level'. They view this as distinct from patient involvement, which refers to 'the involvement of individual patients, together with health professionals, in making decisions about their own health care'. A further issue relates to determining who may be deemed appropriate representatives of the public, as 'lay people' and those able to represent the views of the 'general' public. (For a further discussion of public involvement, *see* Nolte and Wait, in press; Wait and Nolte, in press.)

Although input from the public is sought, how this input is integrated into decision-making remains a rather opaque process. Furthermore, as currently organised, these arrangements reinforce fragmentation of the system because they are attached to individual NHS organisations, rather than crossing boundaries.

This leads to an important question regarding whether public involvement actually creates shifts in governance within healthcare systems. Rowe and Shephard (2002) suggest that public involvement is an instrument to inform decision-making rather than a process that actually devolves power to local communities. Governments may use public involvement initiatives to contain criticism and unrest, thereby deflecting 'political heat' and giving legitimacy to otherwise unpopular policy decisions, especially in the field of rationing (Church *et al.*, 2002; Lupton *et al.*, 1997; Redden, 1999). There is evidence, however, that some public involvement models have evolved away from the 'top-down, paternalistic efforts to extract information from participants' of the past (Abelson *et al.*, 2004; Farrell, 2004; Nolte and Wait, in press). The success of public involvement is contingent on policy-makers' genuine willingness to yield power to the public and the public's genuine engagement in the health policy process. Many public involvement initiatives have been criticised for assigning to the public a reactive rather than a proactive role. Ultimately, managers and policymakers still hold the power to decide how to incorporate the public's input into decision-making in the NHS (Milewa *et al.*, 2002; Wait and Nolte, in press).

Too often public involvement policies are implemented without an explicit evaluative framework, thus precluding the possibility of assessing their impact or

---

[9] For example, Patient and Public Involvement Forums replacing Community Health Councils, and making public involvement statutory in section 11 of the Health and Social Care Act of 2001.

[10] In an editorial for the *British Medical Journal*, Professor Klein of the London School of Economics said he believed Foundation Hospitals have been greeted by 'a wave of apathy from the public and their own staff' and that government plans to involve local people in the running of the hospitals have so far 'largely failed'. In his article, he cites the case of Bradford Teaching Hospital NHS Trust where less than 1% of the population voted for the governors (Klein, 2004).

achievement of desired objectives (Nolte and Wait, in press). For example, Crawford *et al.* (2002) conducted a systematic review of 337 studies of public involvement and found that only 42 studies (12%) reported the effects of involving patients in the development and planning of healthcare. They found that involving patients did contribute to changes in the provision of a range of services, although the effect of involvement strategies on the quality and effectiveness of services was more difficult to ascertain (Crawford *et al.*, 2002). Cayton (2004) has asked '[are we] engaged in a radical rethinking of the relationship between health care providers and the people who pay for them or are we just trying to use patient [and public] compliance to manage the system better?'

Individual responsibility, the nanny state[11] and public health

In his review of UK health, Wanless (2002) introduced the idea of the 'fully-engaged patient', one who undertook 'health-seeking behaviour' and spent more time with a GP but less time actually ill. Full-engagement, according to Wanless, is also associated with lower healthcare costs overall. Again, there is a moral imperative and a pragmatic one. There are two distinct aspects to full-engagement: disease management and prevention.

Least problematic for the state is the accumulating evidence that a patient's engagement in the management of their own condition produces positive outcomes. The role of self-care in future UK health is considered in more detail in Chapters 2 and 3. For the state, however, this creates an incidental issue of boundaries and entitlements in terms of what counts as healthcare, social care, self-care, what kind of support is available to the self-carer and the informal carer, and who pays for what. This is especially relevant in the current English context.

The issue of prevention is politically more problematic. The fully-engaged patient will be expected to take more responsibility for maintaining their health, and the role of government will be conceived mainly in terms of addressing information deficit (DH, 2003; Kennedy, 2003; NHS, 2004) and building health literacy.[12] Libertarians would argue that this is only proper – individuals should have the freedom to pursue their own lives without interference from the state, as long as their actions do not harm others and resist the development of the 'nanny state'.[13]

---

[11] Some question the negative connotations of the 'nanny' (Ashley, 2004) arguing that not all individuals are in the same social position to use information and act upon it, so some will need more help. In particular, it is affluent households who have freedom of choice as well as freedom to deal with the consequences of poor choice. Those who need help with debt, poor housing and poor diet may not see the 'nanny' in quite the same way. This is an empirical question about values and experiences. What is more, Navarro and Shi (2001) compared OECD countries, and found that 'political traditions more committed to distributive policies (both economic and social) and full-employment policies ... were generally more successful in improving the health of populations'.

[12] Health literacy can be defined as 'the degree in which individuals have the capacity to obtain, process, and understand the basic health information and services needed to make appropriate health decisions' (IOM, 2003).

[13] This debate can be reproduced in the entitlement to healthcare. It has already been noted that UK citizens have the right to healthcare free at the point of delivery. This is largely supported by the political elites and the citizenry, but arguments can be made for the 'rolling back'

Hill (1996) argues that it is legitimate for citizens to expect states to play a role in their health, but the state can hold individuals accountable for life-threatening behaviour, and protect society from incurring the consequences of others' behaviour. The state has the right to hold its citizens accountable when they face the consequences of their irresponsible behaviour. A Civitas paper (Bosanquet *et al.*, 2003) also makes a distinction between ill health that is unfortunate and ill health that results from 'irresponsible' behaviour. In terms of entitlement, it can be argued that UK citizens pay taxes and receive healthcare in return. Indeed, it is through social rights that the UK public define their citizenship (Conover *et al.*, 1991). Paton (2000), for example, argues that the tax-funded NHS relieves employers of any obligation to contribute to the healthcare of their workers, and Lister (2005) notes an absence of occupational health services in the UK.

Yet, an individual's health is not only an individual concern. It has ramifications for wider social networks and societies, both in terms of the costs of disease and the risk of infection (hence concerns about parents choosing not to have their children given the MMR vaccine). Nor is health exclusively about individual choice, but partly predicated upon community circumstances, for example, pollution and food preparation. Individual choice can be tightly constrained by powerful commercial interests or by circumstances of employment.

If UK governments are serious about improving health and meeting health targets (DH, 2000; 2004a), they need to be prepared to embark on more comprehensive strategies. The determinants of health are complex and varied (Monaghan *et al.*, 2003) and unevenly distributed across societies. (For more discussion, *see* Determinants of health in Chapter 9.) Individuals face different incentive structures (Halpern and Cockayne, 2004) and governments face conflicts. Health promotion, for instance, is not the only role of the state: for departments of government responsible for economic growth and employment, the manufacture and sales of tobacco (ASH, 2004), alcohol (Institute of Alcohol Studies, 2003; Prime Minister's Strategy Unit, 2004) and food, are beneficial. Typically, UK governments have been reluctant to introduce advertising bans, or to impose some product specifications if the item is legally available. Weak regulation is usually justified in terms of being appropriately liberal, but may also reflect the influence of commercial interests over public policy.

Protecting consumers from food-borne illness is politically unproblematic, and any government not undertaking such arrangements would be considered remiss. Yet, around 50–60 people a year die from food poisoning (Food Standards Agency, 2000). Somehow the inspection of meat is not a violation of libertarian values, yet the regulation of ready meals is. Similarly, it is estimated that 2115 people died from illegal drugs in 1997 compared with 5500 from alcohol in 2000 (ONS, 2004b). In addition, libertarian arguments possibly overstate 'lifestyle' factors in health status. The physical environment, social policy, housing, transport and education are all relevant to health (Yach, 2005).

Arguably governments should be prepared to act on behalf of their citizenry, because 'without minimum levels of health, people cannot fully engage in social

---

of state-provided healthcare in order to provide better incentives to individuals to guard their own health. Socialised medicine, it is argued, spreads the risk, allowing feckless individuals to free-ride, whilst imposing constraints on the freedom of other citizens.

interactions, participate in the political process, exercise the rights of citizenship, generate wealth, create art, and provide for the common security' (Gostin and Bloche, 2003). If the key question is how the state can contribute to better health and wellbeing for its citizens, states need to be prepared to do some rethinking. They face two difficult issues: first deciding where to draw the line on state versus personal responsibility[14] and second which tools to employ in the latter case[15] (Abel-Smith, 1994; Gostin and Bloche, 2003; Wanless, 2003). Selection of policy tools has to be sensitive to individual circumstance and psychology (Halpern *et al.*, 2004). Different attitudes towards the future risks and 'deferred gratification', for example, can be extremely important in a health context, particularly when trying to change present behaviour to effect future health benefits (for example, forgoing smoking to avoid a heart attack in the future).

It is questionable whether a key role of the state is to provide a countervailing force to individualism and consumerism (which is not to argue that people should tolerate poor quality services at the whim of unaccountable providers) and to support a return to the more collectivist attitudes of the past (Pierre and Peters, 2000). The NHS – which forms such a central role in national consciousness – might be a vehicle in which increasingly different populations are brought together in common endeavour, with the possibility that health policy could be reconfigured to support coherence and equity.

Public health law

There are additional concerns regarding the inadequacy of current public health laws (Monaghan *et al.*, 2003). Article 11 of the European Social Chapter requires states to 'remove the causes of illness, prevent disease and advise citizens on how to look after their health' (Montgomery, 2003). The post of Under Secretary of State for Public Health was first created in 1998.[16] The interpretation of this function has been fairly open, with a role for local authorities who 'provide a variety of environmental health services aimed at protecting public health, ranging from pest control and noise pollution to the inspection and registration of food premises. Other local authority responsibilities such as housing, education, waste disposal, and the provision of sport and leisure facilities also have the potential to make a major contribution to UK health' (Yach, 2005). Despite its long history (Montgomery, 2003), there are still concerns that current public health legislation is inadequate, with no clear duties or specific responsibilities (Monaghan *et al.*, 2003).

---

[14] These include fiscal and monetary interventions (incentives and subsidies), regulation, direct provision, participatory guarantees, R&D, information and education (Milo, 1986, quoted in Abel-Smith, 1994).

[15] Power to tax and spend, power to alter the informational environment, power to alter the built environment, power to alter the socio-economic environment, direct regulation of persons, professionals, and businesses, indirect regulation through the tort system, deregulation: law as a barrier to health (for example, laws restricting the sale or provision of syringes and needles).

[16] The Under Secretary of State for Public Health as specified in 1998 is responsible for cancer, coronary heart disease, tobacco policy, communicable diseases, immunisation, health inequalities, drug and alcohol misuse, and sexual health issues.

Under the European Social Charter, the UK state is obliged to provide care for the sick who are unable to provide care for themselves. 'This commitment does not require states to provide a comprehensive health service, as it only covers the treatment of illness, not health promotion, and extends only to those unable to purchase care privately' (Montgomery, 2003). Predating the European Social Charter, and only relevant to healthcare services, is the National Health Service Act of 1997 under which the Secretary of State for Health is bound 'to continue the promotion in England and Wales [Scotland has a separate Act] of a comprehensive health service ... and, for that purpose to provide or secure the effective services in accordance with this Act', ensuring the provision of, though not necessarily providing, services they deem 'appropriate', 'necessary' and 'reasonable' (McLean and Mason, 2003). For further discussion on public health, *see* Chapter 3.

Conclusions

Pierre and Peters (2000) note that systems of governance always change. In general, states in the UK are making less use of coercive policy instruments, are deliberately courting and cultivating the private market, have restructured their own institutions to produce 'arm's-length' agencies and quangos, and have separated the policy and operational functions (Winstanley *et al.*, 1995). In turn, this has created a greater need for regulation and control, undermining traditional accountabilities (Day and Klein, 1987; O'Neill, 2002). The embedded role of the state in UK health policy is firmly established and likely to remain in the future.

Health policy involves choice between conflicting goods – two desirable but mutually exclusive choices. Trade-off decisions will always present themselves between the need to support economic growth and yet control healthcare spending, or the need to support the autonomy of citizens and yet protect a population's health. These questions go to the heart of the question of what sort of democratic society we wish to inhabit. There will always be a role for the state and elected politicians in health. The state will always have relations with players in markets, professional experts, devolved jurisdictions and citizens.

This chapter has discussed the emergence of the policy context of the UK and where it may be headed. Although much debate will depend on political persuasion, there is one vital area for development which is up to central government: to be steadfast in holding a focus on a system of health, rather than a health (care) system (Yach, 2005). This alone will create a huge agenda for bold choices and trade-offs between the parties discussed in this chapter.

Policy recommendations

- The state should acknowledge it does and should provide a broad and values-based policy context for health as most of the risks to health fall outside the healthcare system.
- The state has a key role in setting the 'health' agenda beyond ensuring the provision of healthcare as cost-effectively as possible.
- Not everyone will become expert patients and literate in health, which will influence individual health status and needs to be addressed in policy.

- Commitment to market-based values as a basis for policymaking in a public healthcare system should be reviewed, particularly as this is associated with a social trend to move away from political, and, debatably, civic engagement.
- There needs to be greater clarification of the state's role in regulating the practice of doctors, including education and training.
- Regulation needs to be anchored within a robust system of intelligence designed to inform individuals and organisations with an interest in the performance of the system.
- A regulatory framework should look to the long term, and address:
  - individual choice and community and population concerns
  - the tax-funded system accountable to public and patients
  - the performance of healthcare professionals
  - the mixed economy of public and private sector providers.
- Mechanisms need to be developed for public involvement to address the accountability of the individual within the state system as well as any 'democratic deficit'.
- Real choice will depend on good patient information and the reduction of dependency on providers.
- Greater focus on individual responsibility raises questions about the role of the state in providing information to enable individual choice and in embracing policies to protect or promote health.
- More funding and time should be given to assessing the effectiveness of public health interventions and innovation projects, such as ensuring that the state has the power to protect the health of the public.

References

Abel-Smith B (1994) Planning health policy. In: *An Introduction to Health: policy, planning, and financing*. Longman Publishing, New York, pp. 47–62.

Abelson J, Forest P-G, Eyles J, Casebeer A, Mackean G and Effective Public Consultation Project Team (2004) Will it make a difference if I show up and share? A citizens' perspective on improving public involvement processes for health system decision-making. *Journal of Health Services Research & Policy*. 9(4): 205–12.

Appleby J and Dixon J (2004) Patient choice in the NHS. *British Medical Journal*. **329**: 61–2.

ASH (2004) Factsheet no. 18. The tobacco industry. http://www.ash.org.uk/html/factsheets/html/fact18.html. Accessed: 21 April 2004.

Ashley J (2004) Britain needs the nanny state now more than ever. *The Guardian*. 1.1.04.

Baggott R (1998) Care in the community. In: *Health and Healthcare in Britain*. Macmillan Press Ltd, London, pp. 228–47.

Baggott R (2004) *Health and Health Care in Britain*. Palgrave Macmillan, Basingstoke.

Bambra C, Fox D and Scott-Samuel A (2003) *Towards a New Politics of Health*. Politics of Health Group, University of Liverpool, Liverpool.

BBC (2004a) Guide: How the healthcare system works in England. http://www.bbc.co.uk/dna/ican/A2454978. Accessed: 20 May 2004.

BBC (2004b) Guide: How the healthcare system works in Northern Ireland. http://www.bbc.co.uk/dna/ican/A2494181. Accessed: 20 May 2004.

BBC (2004c) Guide: How the healthcare system works in Scotland. http://www.bbc.co.uk/dna/ican/A2459388. Accessed: 20 May 2004.

BBC (2004d) Guide: How the healthcare system works in Wales. http://www.bbc.co.uk/dna/ican/ A2455472. Accessed: 20 May 2004.

Bentley JM and Nash DB (1998) How Pennsylvania hospitals have responded to publicly released reports on coronary artery bypass graft surgery. *Joint Commission Journal on Quality Improvement.* **24**(1): 40–9.

BMA (2003) Ethics brief. Issue 67, October 2003: Right to treatment in other European countries. http://www.bma.org.uk/ap.nsf/Content/EthicsBrief67. Accessed: 31 March 2005.

BMA (2004) *Health Policy Debate: May 2004.* British Medical Association, London.

Bosanquet N, Browne A, Bull A, Day G, Desai M, Disney H, Green DG, Irvine B, Lea R, Lees C, Neil A, Ormerod P, Pollard S, Smith S and Young M (2003) *The Final Report of the Health Policy Consensus Group: a new consensus for NHS reform.* Civitas, London.

Cayton H (2004) *Patient Engagement and Patient Decision-making in England.* Improving Quality of Health Care in the United States and the United Kingdom: strategies for change and action. 11–13 July 2003. The Commonwealth Fund, Pennyhill Park, UK.

Church J, Saunders M, Wanke M, Pong R, Spooner C and Dorgan M (2002) Citizen participation in health decision-making: past experience and future prospects. *Journal of Public Health Policy.* **23**: 12–32.

Clarke J (2004) *A Consuming Public?* Lecture in ESRC/AHRB Cultures of Consumption Series, Royal Society, 22 April 2004. The Open University, 16, London.

Clarke J and Newman J (1997) *The Managerial State.* Sage, London.

Conover PJ, Crewe IM and Searing DD (1991) The nature of citizenship in the United States and Great Britain: empirical comments on theoretical themes. *Journal of Politics.* **53**(3): 800–32.

Conservative Party (2005) Speech to Conservative Party Conference, 2004. http://www.conservatives.com/tile.do?def=news.story.page&obj_id=116324&speeches=1. Accessed: 29 March 2005.

Crawford MJ, Rutter C, Manley T, Weaver K, Bhui N, Fulop N and Tyrer P (2002) Systematic review of involving patients in the planning and development of healthcare. *British Medical Journal.* **325**: 1263–7.

Dawson S and Sausman C (2005) *Future Health Organisations and Systems.* Palgrave Macmillan, Basingstoke.

Day P and Klein R (1987) *Accountabilities in Five Public Services.* Tavistock Publications, London.

Dean M (2004) Delegates at the Labour conference must challenge health policy. *The Guardian.* 29.9.04.

Degeling P, Maxwell S, Macbeth F, Kennedy J and Coyle B (2003) The impact of CHI: some evidence from Wales. *Quality in Primary Care.* **11**: 147–57.

Department of Trade and Industry (2003) *Bioscience 2015. Improving National Health, Increasing National Wealth.* Department of Trade and Industry, Bioscience Innovation and Growth Team, London.

Dewar S (2003) *Government and the NHS: time for a new relationship.* King's Fund, London.

DH (2000) *The NHS Plan: a plan for investment, a plan for reform. Cmnd 4818–I.* Department of Health, London.

DH (2002) *Shifting the Balance of Power: the next steps.* Department of Health, London.

DH (2003) *The Expert Patient: a new approach to chronic disease management for the 21st Century.* Department of Health, London.

DH (2004a) *Choosing Health: making healthier choices easier. Cmnd 6374.* London, Department of Health.

DH (2004b) *NHS Improvement Plan: putting people at the heart of public services.* Department of Health, London.

Donaldson C and Gerard K (1989) Countering moral hazard in public and private healthcare systems: a review of recent evidence. *Journal of Social Policy*. **18**(2): 235–51.

Donelly L (2004) The end is CHI. *Health Service Journal*. **114**.

Dunleavy P and O'Leary B (1987) *Theories of the State: the politics of liberal democracy*. Macmillan Education, London.

Engel GL (1981) The need for a new medical model: a challenge to bio-medicine. In: AL Kaplan, HT Engelhardt and JJ McCartney (eds) *Concepts of Health and Disease: interdisciplinary perspectives*. Addison Wesley, London.

Enthoven A (1985) *Reflections on the Management of the NHS*. Nuffield Provincial Hospitals Trust, London.

Farrell C (2004) *Patient and Public Involvement in Health: the evidence for policy implementation*. Department of Health, London.

Florin D and Dixon J (2004) Public involvement in healthcare. *British Medical Journal*. **328**: 159–61.

Food Standards Agency (2000) Food Standards Agency to reduce food poisoning by 20%. http://www.food.gov.uk/news/pressreleases/2000/jul/reducefoodpoisoning. Accessed: 1 April 2005.

Gostin LO and Bloche MG (2003) The politics of public health: a reply to Richard Epstein. *Perspectives in Biology and Medicine*. **46**(S3): S160–75.

Greener I (2003) Patient choice in the NHS: the view from economic sociology. *Social Theory & Health*. **1**: 72–89.

Greener I (2004) The three moments of New Labour's health policy discourse. *Policy and Politics*. **32**(3): 303–16.

Greer S (2005) Personal communication.

Greer S (2004) *Four Way Bet: how devolution has led to four different models for the NHS*. University College London, London.

Halpern D, Bates C, Beales G and Heathfield A (2004) *Personal Responsibility and Changing Behaviour: the state of knowledge and its implications for public policy*. Prime Minister's Strategy Unit, London.

Halpern D and Cockayne A (2004) *Trust, engagement and legitimacy in public institutions. Summary of interim Analytical Report*. Cabinet Office, London.

Ham C and Alberti KGMM (2002) The medical profession, the public, and the government. *British Medical Journal*. **324**: 838–42.

Harper R (2002) *Trends in Social Capital*. Prime Minister's Strategy Unit, Strategic Futures, Social Capital, Office for National Statistics, London.

Harrison S and Ahmed W (2000) Medical Autonomy and the UK State 1975 to 2025. *Sociology*. **34**(1): 129–46.

Hawkes N (2004) Private medicine looks for pick-me-up. *The Times*. 11.6.04.

Hibbard J, Sofaer S and Jewett J (1996) Condition-specific performance information: assessing salience, comprehension and approaches for communicating quality. *Health Care Financing Review*. **18**(1): 95–109.

Hibbard JH and Jewett JJ (1997) Will quality report cards help? *Health Affairs*. **16**(3): 218–28.

Higgins J and Wiles R (1992) Study of patients who chose private healthcare for treatment. *Journal of General Practice*. **42**: 326–9.

Hill TP (1996) Health care: a social contract in transition. *Social Science and Medicine*. **43**(5): 783–9.

HM Treasury (2003) *Lambert Review of Business–University Collaboration. Final Report*. HM Treasury, London.

HSJ (2004) Goodbye to all that. *Health Service Journal*. **114**: 16–19.

Hutton W (2000) *New Life for Health: The Commission on the NHS*. Vintage, London.

Institute of Alcohol Studies (2003) Economic Costs and Benefits. Social Costs of Alcohol. http://216.239.59.104/search?q=cache:VaK4uknRaJ8J:www.ias.org.uk/factsheets/costs-benefits.pdf+Economic+Costs+and+Benefits.+Social+Costs+of+Alcohol&hl=en. Accessed: 29 March 2005.

IOM (2003) *Informing the Future: critical issues in health.* Institute of Medicine, Washington DC.

Kavanaugh T (2004) Health factories 'cure NHS'. *The Sun.* 10.5.04.

Kennedy I (2003) Patients are experts in their own field. *British Medical Journal.* **326**: 1276–7.

King's Fund (2002) *The Future of the National Health Service: a framework for debate.* King's Fund, London.

Klein R (2004) The first wave of NHS foundation trusts. *British Medical Journal.* **328**: 1332.

Klein R (2005) The public–private mix in the UK. In: A Maynard (ed.) *The Public–Private Mix for Health.* Radcliffe Publishing, pp. 41–60.

Leatherman S and Sutherland K (2003) *The Quest for Quality in the NHS: a mid-term evaluation of the ten-year quality agenda.* TSO, London.

Leatherman S and Sutherland K (2005) *The Quest for Quality in the NHS: a chartbook on quality of care in the UK.* Radcliffe Publishing, Oxford.

Lister G (2005) Health Policy Futures and Cost Scenarios for England 2003–2023. In: S Dawson and C Sausman (eds) *Future Health Organisations and Systems.* Palgrave Macmillan, Basingstoke.

Lupton C, Peckham S and Taylor P (1997) *Managing Public Involvement in Healthcare Purchasing.* Open University Press, Buckingham.

Lynch J, Due P, Muntaner C and Smith GD (2000) Social capital – is it a good investment strategy for public health? *Journal of Epidemiology and Community Health.* **54**(404): 404–8.

Marshall TH (1963) *Class, Citizenship, and Social Development.* Greenwood Publishing Group, Westport, CT.

Maynard A (2005) *The Public–Private Mix for Health.* Radcliffe Publishing, Oxford.

McKeown T (1979) *The role of medicine.* Basil Blackwell, Oxford.

McLean S and Mason JK (2003) *Legal & Ethical Aspects of Healthcare.* Greenwich Medical Media, London.

Mennemeyer S, Morrisey M and Howard L (1997) Death and reputation: how consumers acted upon HCFA information. *Inquiry.* **34**: 117–28.

Milewa T, Dowswell G and Harrison S (2002) Partnerships, power and the 'new' politics of community participation in British healthcare. *Social Policy and Administration.* **36**: 796–809.

Monaghan S, Huws D and Navarro M (2003) *The Case for a New UK Health of the People Act.* The Nuffield Trust, London.

Montgomery J (2003) Public health law. In: *Public Health.* Oxford University Press, Oxford, pp. 23–50.

MORI (2004) Attitudes to public services reform. http://www.mori.com/polls/2004/radio4-today.shtml. Accessed: 18 October 2004.

Mulligan J and Appleby J (2001) The NHS and Labour's battle for public opinion. In: A Park, J Curtice, K Thomson and C Bromley (eds) *British Social Attitudes: the 18th Report – public bodies, social ties.* Sage, London.

Mythen M and Coffey T (2004) *Patient Power: the impact of patient choice on the future NHS.* The New Health Network, London.

Navarro V and Shi L (2001) The political context of social inequalities and health. *Social Science and Medicine.* **52**: 481–91.

NCC (2004) *Making Public Services Personal: a new compact for public services.* National Consumer Council, London.

Nettleton S (1995) *The Sociology of Health & Illness.* Polity Press, London.

Newman J (2001) *Modernising Governance: new labour, policy and society.* Sage, London.

NHS (2004) Expert Patients Programme. http://www.expertpatients.nhs.uk/index.shtml. Accessed: 3 October 2004.

Nolte E and Wait S. Enhancing responsiveness in healthcare: the role of public involvement. *Health Economics, Policy and Law*. In press.

O'Neill O (2002) *Reith lectures 2002: A question of trust*. http://www.bbc.co.uk/radio4/reith2002/lecture4.shtml. Accessed: 3 October 2004.

Office of Public Services Reform (2002) *Reforming Our Public Services*. Office of Public Services Reform, London.

ONS (2004a) *Paper 1: Public Service Productivity*. http://www.statistics.gov.uk/cci/article.asp?id=987. Accessed: 29 March 2005.

ONS (2004b) *Social Trends 34: A portrait of British society*. http://www.statistics.gov.uk/pdfdir/sot0104.pdf. Accessed: 21 October 2004.

OUP (1999) *Oxford Concise English Dictionary*. Oxford University Press, Oxford.

Page B (2004) What they really really want. *Health Service Journal*. **114**: 16–19.

Paton C (2000) *World, Class, Britain: political economy, political theory and British politics*. Macmillan, London.

Pierre J and Peters BG (2000) *Governance, Politics and the State*. Macmillan, Basingstoke.

Pollock AM, Shaoul J and Vickers N (2002) Private finance and 'value for money' in NHS hospitals: a policy in search of a rationale? *British Medical Journal*. **324**: 1205–9.

Power M (1994) *The Audit Explosion*. Demos, London.

Power M (1997) *The Audit Society: rituals of verification*. Oxford University Press, Oxford.

Prime Minister's Strategy Unit (2004) *Alcohol Harm Reduction Strategy For England*. Cabinet Office, London.

Redden CJ (1999) Rationing care in the community: engaging citizens in health care decision making. *Journal of Health Politics, Policy and Law*. **24**: 1363–89.

Reid J (2005) *Limits of the Market, Constraints of the State: the public good and the NHS*. The Social Market Foundation, London.

Rhodes R (1996) The new governance: governing without government. *Political Studies*. **44**(4): 652–68.

Rice JA (1995) *Toward Public–Private Mix for Health Gain*. Lakeland Color Press, Minneapolis.

Robinson S and Brodie M (1997) Understanding the quality challenge for health consumers: the kaiser/AHCPR survey. *Journal on Quality Improvement*. **23**(5): 239–44.

Rothstein B (2004) *The Universal Welfare State and Social Capital*. Fifth European Conference on Health Economics. London School of Economics, London.

Rowe R and Shepherd M (2002) Public participation in the new NHS: closer to citizen control? *Social Policy and Administration*. **36**(3): 275–90.

Rushmer M and Hallam A (2004) *Mental Health Law Research Programme. Analysis of reponses to consultation*. Scottish Executive Social Research, Edinburgh.

Scally G and Donaldson LJ (1998) Looking forward: clinical governance and the drive for quality improvement in the new NHS in England. *British Medical Journal*. **317**: 61–5.

Schneider EC and Epstein AM (1998) Use of public performance reports. *Journal of American Medical Administration*. **279**(20): 1638–42.

Smee C (1995) Self-governing trusts and GP fundholders: the British experience. In: R Saltman and C von Otter (eds) *Implementing Planned Markets in Health Care*. Open University Press, Buckingham.

Stevens S (2004) Reform strategies for the English NHS. *Health Affairs*. **23**(3): 37–44.

The Economist (2004). Got a match? http://www.economist.com/displaystory.cfm?story_id=3432570. Accessed: 31 March 2005.

Timmins N (2004) Consultants to resist big fee cuts for private operations. *Financial Times*. 11.6.04.

Vaiana ME and McGlynn EA (2002) What cognitive science tells us about the design of reports for consumers. *Medical Care Research and Review*. **59**(1): 3–35.

Wait S and Nolte E. Benchmarking health systems: trends, conceptual issues and future perspectives. *Benchmarking International Journal*. **12**(4/5). In press.

Walshe K (2002) The rise of regulation in the NHS. *British Medical Journal*. **324**: 967–70.

Wanless D (2001) *Securing our Future Health: taking a long-term view. Interim report*. HM Treasury, London.

Wanless D (2002) *Securing our Future Health: taking a long-term view*. HM Treasury, London.

Wanless D (2003) *Securing Good Health for the Whole Population: population health trends*. HM Treasury, London.

White K (1991) The sociology of health and illness. *Current Sociology*. **39**(2): 1–82.

Williams A (2005) The pervasive role of ideology in the optimisation of the public–private mix in public healthcare systems. In: A Maynard (ed.) *The Public–Private Mix for Health*. Radcliffe Publishing, Oxford.

Winstanley D, Sorabji D and Dawson S (1995) When the pieces don't fit: a stakeholder power matrix to analyse public sector restructuring. *Public Money & Management*. **15**(2): 19–26.

Yach D (2005) A system for health or a health care system? In: S Dawson and C Dargie (eds) *Future Health Organisations and Systems*. Palgrave, Cambridge.

Chapter 5

Who's going to care?

Linda Rosenstrøm Chang, Alison Kitson and Alison Petch

The provision of care and possible future developments and challenges to provision are explored in this chapter. It begins with a discussion of human resources, and asks whether the UK can satisfy the growing demand for carers. It examines different types of carers: self-carers, informal carers and professional carers. It considers health and social care policy, and its implications for carer roles in society.

The working definition proposed to encompass all these forms of care is 'helping an individual with the respectful interaction between the person needing and the person giving support'. It assumes that the type of care being delivered will meet certain basic values with regard to respect, dignity, privacy, safety and involvement (Kendall, 2001). Individuals expect professional care when their needs for care extend beyond their own or informal carers' ability to deliver it.

Within a health and disease context, there are many different kinds of care. Some definitions refer to location, whether within a hospital setting under professional care, under the auspices of the GP's expanded facilities, or in the 'one-stop health shop' (Davies, 2003). Others refer to the identity of the carer, whether a self-carer, informal carer or professional carer. A third group refer to the duration of care or the stage of illness at which care is given, so may refer to long-term, residential or palliative care. There may be an overlap between categories.[1]

The shortage of healthcare and social care staff poses an immense challenge.[2] The demand for care is evident in Chapters 1 and 4, both of which raise the issues of the ageing population and the implications of chronic disease and mental illnesses. This challenge will necessitate a redrawing of the boundaries around care.[3] First, the support needed to optimise the individual's self-care capability should be taken into consideration: the skills, information, knowledge and additional resources needed to lead better, healthier lives. Second, consideration needs to be given to optimising independence and wellbeing when self-care ability fails. This may take the form of a regular discussion with a community pharmacist or nurse, a check-up with the local GP or trauma surgery. These are all aspects of the 'care continuum' (*see* Figure 2).

---

[1] Some examples of care are: self, personal, home, community, emergency, immediate, intermediate, long-term, supportive, nursing, social, hospice and end-of-life, palliative, alternative and integrated.

[2] This workforce is, like the population overall, ageing, yet it is predicted that 300 000 more healthcare staff will be needed over the next 20 years – 62 000 more doctors, 108 000 more nurses and 45 000 more therapists and scientists (Wanless, 2002).

[3] The boundaries are shifting between primary, secondary and tertiary care. This will impact upon traditional professional roles and fundamentally on how services are funded.

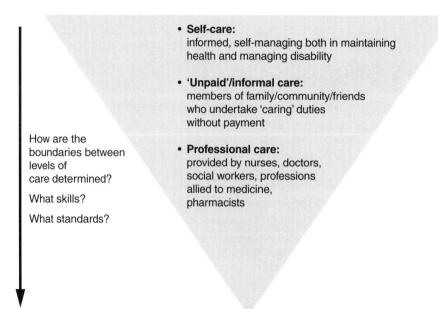

How are the
boundaries between
levels of
care determined?

What skills?

What standards?

• **Self-care:**
informed, self-managing both in maintaining
health and managing disability

• **'Unpaid'/informal care:**
members of family/community/friends
who undertake 'caring' duties
without payment

• **Professional care:**
provided by nurses, doctors,
social workers, professions
allied to medicine,
pharmacists

Figure 2   Redefining care.

Scarce human resources

In this section, carer roles are examined and pressures on the sector, particularly retention and recruitment, are raised. Recent years have seen frequent restructuring of the healthcare system in search of greater control, more patient-centred care, or greater value for money (DH, 1997; 2001; 2004a). These changes should be continually evaluated in terms of cost-efficiency and quality. Further research into how restructuring is working should take place before more changes are made.

Self-care

The Wanless reports (2002; 2004) propose maximising the individual's self-care[4] potential throughout their life, thereby reducing the need for informal, paid or professional care. Further analysis is required regarding how this would work alongside the investment in prevention, health promotion and educational interventions. Self-diagnostic tools for the training of practitioners have been suggested (DH, 2005b) although not everyone will be capable of caring for themselves.

Learning how to self-care will require changes across education and healthcare systems, with more emphasis being placed on basics such as personal health and

---

[4] Care administered by the individual suffering disease, such as self-medication or self-checks (Wanless, 2004). Interestingly, a wider definition is suggested by the DH in a recent paper on self-care: '[self-care] is the care taken by individuals towards their own health and wellbeing, and includes the care extended to their children, family, friends and others in neighbourhoods and local communities' (DH, 2005b). This definition includes informal care which it classifies as self-care.

wellbeing, effective parenting and child care, fitness and nutrition. As access to information on disease management increases, so self-care will extend to the effective and on-going management of chronic illnesses. Policy initiatives demonstrate that the NHS (2004) would prefer individuals to be in control of their own disease management (*see also* CPPIH, 2004).

As the individual's self-care potential changes, their boundaries with other carers will be redrawn. Wider issues, for example equality of access to information and support (and recognition that some groups may be less equipped to self-care), will require policy interventions. An underlying assumption is that individuals prefer to take care of themselves and that health and social policy priorities are to assist with requisite support mechanisms when self-care starts to fail. An issue to consider when trying to maximise the potential of self-care, is how self-care will safeguard the most disadvantaged people. This is an important question, particularly in the light of current government debates around reducing maintenance support benefits and encouraging people with long-term medical conditions back to work (Johnson, 2004; MENCAP, 2005).

Unpaid/informal care

Between self-care and more formal health and social support, there is a significant growing number of unpaid or informal carers. Meeting demand for long-term care is highly dependent on the supply of informal care.

The Personal Social Services Research Unit (PSSRU) has estimated the number of older people dependent on informal care could rise from 2.5 million to just over 4 million by 2020 (PSSRU, 2003a). It is predicted that there will be more spouse carers too (PSSRU, 2003a). Even with informal carers, long-term care expenditure could grow between 108–151%, depending on the life expectancy of older people (PSSRU, 2003a).

PSSRU has sought to predict the number of people who will report long-standing limiting illness, assuming illness rates remain the same. They suggest there could be a rise from 6.42 million in 1991 to 10.2 million in 2037 and, while there are difficulties in estimating the numbers of people with limiting illness, the figures indicate that the need for informal carers is not declining (PSSRU, 2003a). The number of carers could correspondingly rise from approximately 6 million to 9.1 million in 2037 (PSSRU, 2003a), depending on where the locus for care lies. For instance, it may be that the state will provide more formal care in which case the need for informal carers would lessen.

It is estimated that there are 16 million 'informal carers', representing the equivalent of 1.7 million full-time employed care-givers, who perform a range of tasks such as shopping, cleaning, washing, administering medication and treating pressure sores (Henwood, 2001).

It is estimated that one in five people will become a carer during their lifetime (Carers UK, 2002). A woman has a 50:50 likelihood of becoming a carer by the time she is 59, while a man reaches the same odds at the age of 74 (Carers UK, 2002). It is estimated that 301 000 people become carers every year. According to one estimate, this figure represents an annual value of £57.4 billion (Carers UK, 2002). Over a ten-year period, from 1985–95, the proportion of carers providing more intensive care (in terms of hours) has increased (Carers UK, 2002). New research has estimated that more than one million young people (aged 7–19) may be involved in caring roles (Princess Royal Trust for Carers, 2004).

If the ratio of carer to cared-for remains the same, there could be a shortfall of informal carers (BBC, 2004a). If only a small percentage of carers was to give up caring, the impact would be significant in economic terms (PSSRU, 2003a). The effect of such a decline would depend on the extent to which residential and home care substitutes for informal care. At present, the health and social care system is very much dependent on the efforts of the informal carers. Given future estimates, it is likely that the demand for informal support will also outstrip supply. If people have to work longer hours and more years to contribute to the economy, they will have less time to be informal carers and they may not choose to be carers. One policy response would be to provide more state support to adults and young people caring for their elderly dependent relatives, in the manner that childcare is currently provided.

The implications of the growing role of informal carers are worrying. Morbidity in one spouse can contribute to morbidity in the other spouse due to the care-giver burden (Christakis, 2004). In a caring arrangement the informal carer will typically place the health needs of the ill person ahead of his or her own requirements (Guberman *et al.*, 2003). As a consequence, two-thirds of unpaid carers providing more than 50 hours of weekly care report that their health has been adversely affected by caring demands (Iles, 2003). Of informal carers, one-tenth of men and one-quarter of women suffer from fatigue (Baggott, 1998). Over half of carers providing substantial amounts of care have been treated for a stress-related disorder and half of the same group has sustained a physical injury since they first started caring (Carers UK, 2002). As a consequence of increased informal care associated with the ageing population, there may be an increase of ill health in the informal carer.

Financial problems associated with caring arrangements also add to the level of stress (Baggott, 1998). After five years of providing substantial amounts of care, the carer's financial situation tends to worsen significantly (Carers UK, 2002). Many carers who have looked after someone for more than ten years are financially disadvantaged, with a third of all informal carers falling into this category (Baggott, 1998). Of carers aged 56 to 60, 78% give up work to care, and therefore become financially worse-off (Carers UK, 2002). There is a direct correlation between the amount of hours informal carers spend on the labour market and their ability to care: the more they informally care, the less likely they are to work and if they work, they earn less and work fewer hours (Carmichael and Charles, 1998).

In recognition of the financial burden of informal care, the Attendance Allowance and the Disability Allowance can be used by a person in need to pay for care (McLean and Mason, 2003). The payment of an allowance to the informal carer legitimates family care but at the same time raises questions about the knowledge and skills of the informal carer (Forbat and Henderson, 2003). The relationship between informal carers and the cared-for is an important factor differentiating informal care from that given in an institutional, professional setting. Since the informal carer by nature is not a formal carer, status and confidentiality issues – how much the formal carer tells the informal carer – can also be a problem between the patient, the informal carer and the formal carer (Forbat and Henderson, 2003). While emotions can complicate the provision of care in some senses, research shows that technically competent treatment without personal connection is less effective (Forbat and Henderson, 2003). Research also shows that hospital-at-home interventions can prolong the overall sickness time, while patient satisfaction is higher (Sibbald *et al.*, 2004).

Social care workforce

Social or healthcare support is required when self-care and the person's need for caring support extends beyond their own or immediate family resources. Depending on the definitions used, there are 1.2 million people employed in delivering social care services in the UK, including local authority social services staff, residential, day and domiciliary care staff and agency workers (General Social Care Council, 2003; *The Guardian*, 2004). Traditional social care roles also include a limited number of NHS staff.[5]

While the need for social carers will increase in the future, the sector is suffering from an ongoing recruitment and retention crisis due to its poor image and low status, linked to low pay and lack of career development opportunities (EOC, 2004). The sector was the 'surprise loser' in the 2004 spending review (Rankin, 2004), which may be an indication of its low policy saliency.

One in nine local authority social services' posts was vacant in 2002–03, while the annual turnover rate was 13%. London has the highest vacancy and turnover rates: up to 39 and 24% respectively (Hutt and Buchan, 2005). In general, turnover is higher among unqualified care workers than social workers, higher in the independent sector than in local authorities and higher among part-time than full-time staff (Eborall and Garmeson, 2001). It is plausible that the shortage of support staff affects the quality, as well as the quantity, of service provision. An investigation has been launched into the future challenges and demands of social care and the findings are expected in Spring 2006 (King's Fund, 2005).

Current and future shortfalls in social carer numbers could be addressed by adopting broad strategies to improve recruitment and retention. The low status attached to caring (Research Works, 2001) must be addressed, so that carers are not denigrated as unskilled and proper levels of training should become a standard element of recruitment. At present, low pay also makes social care work a less attractive option within the UK labour market.

Some local authorities have been successful in recruiting staff by introducing part-time or term-time work, job-sharing, weekend-only contracts, childcare and crèches, annualised hours quotas, 'golden hellos' (BBC, 2004b) and more competitive rates of pay (Eborall and Garmeson, 2001). They have also shown flexibility in terms of hiring care staff with other experience and qualifications and helping unqualified staff pass exams through training programmes (BBC, 2004d).

The retention of social carers also tends to be impeded by the stress, low salaries, time pressure, anti-social work hours and lack of career development. Successful measures to improve retention have included consulting staff in decision-making, adopting an open-door policy and introducing flexible work hours, and creating new posts with skills mixes, secondments, staff development programmes, improved physical working environment, respite periods and career breaks. Reducing

---

[5] Certain definitions of social carer roles also encompass early years childcare, foster carers, a wider range of NHS staff who carry out care work and education assistants in schools.

bureaucracy and maximising user contact have also been effective (Eborall and Garmeson, 2001).

Latest figures show that 80% of the care workforce and 38% of NHS staff have no formal qualifications for their work (EOC, 2004; Rogers, 2002) but by 2008, 50% of the care provided by a domiciliary agency will have to be delivered by NVQ2-qualified staff (DH, 2003). While this may improve the quality of care home staff, it could impede recruitment of staff. There is controversy over whether formal qualifications are useful (PSSRU, 2003b; Rogers, 2002) and concern that older staff will be reluctant to undertake training and may leave the workforce (EOC, 2004).

A clearer understanding of roles within the social care sector is needed, in particular the nature of support staff roles. This would not only improve carers' understanding of how to change roles and advance their careers, but would also improve the image of social care by demonstrating the value and importance of all roles. There needs to be recognition that for many posts there are increasing demands for flexibility and blurring of roles. Guidelines on the provision of NHS continuing care have led to changing boundaries, with much of the support traditionally delivered to older people in long-stay NHS beds being redefined as social care. The government's Green Paper on the reform of social care may be a step in the right direction, although no new money has been committed to this 15-year vision (DH, 2005a).

Nursing workforce

There are more than 500 000 nurses and 130 000 doctors working in the UK (Skills for Health, 2003). Their care roles are likely to be influenced by two key trends over the next decade: the ongoing demand for healthcare support and the continued inability of most western countries to meet the demand. In addition, as policy shifts to investment in organised self-care initiatives (through greater access to information, self-diagnosis and self-management), the role of professional healthcarers will change. Primarily, the trend will be for professionals to become increasingly technical experts and 'quality controllers' of whole systems or pathways of care.

Staff shortages and a rising demand for care means that fewer nurses are having to care for more people (Finlayson et al., 2002b). Wanless (2002) argues that the number of nurses estimated by the NHS Plan (DH, 2000) will match demand. An NHS vacancies survey in 2000 in England suggested there were 10 000 vacancies for registered nurses and midwives, while the Royal College of Nursing estimated there were 22 000 vacancies[6] (Finlayson et al., 2002a). In Scotland, the number of nurses and midwives is increasing, but nursing vacancies are increasing too (Marshall, 2004). The government's goal is to recruit 115 000 more nurses by 2008 (RCN, 2004a), though consideration still needs to be given to utilising nursing time to meet extra demand.

There is a 15% turnover of nurses per year, with a 38% turnover in London (BMA, 2004c; Finlayson et al., 2002a). Factors contributing to the turnover rate

---

[6] The disparity is due to the way vacancies are calculated. The NHS only counts positions that have been vacant for more than three months, while the RCN counts the post as vacant on the day it becomes vacant.

include low pay and high costs of living,[7] rising levels of (early) retirement, the perception that nursing is undervalued in society and the workplace, competition from other employment opportunities,[8] the increasing frequency of career breaks (including maternity and paternity leave), the demands of skills upgrading and retraining, jobs abroad and the experience of racism and violence in the workplace (Finlayson *et al.*, 2002a,b). High turnover results in higher costs and lower morale, and affects the quality of patient care because existing staff spend time familiarising new nurses with the job (BMA, 2004c).

One out of every five nurses on the UK professional register is aged 50 years or older and the mean age of nurses is increasing. With older nurses returning to work and younger nurses not replacing older ones in sufficient numbers, it is likely that one in four working nurses will be aged 50 or older by 2010 (Buchan, 1999; Finlayson *et al.*, 2002a).

The impact of the European Working Time Directive on doctors' hours has a knock-on effect on nursing staff. Skills-mix changes do not necessarily reduce costs, such as with nurse-doctor substitution in primary care, as more resources are needed to deliver the same quality of care (Sibbald *et al.*, 2004).

Several strategies have been suggested to address the shortfall of nurses. These include better retention of the healthcare sector of the existing workforce, attracting younger cohorts into nursing, changing practices, organising work to maximise use of time and recruiting more nurses from abroad.

Assessing the professional development and employment needs of the growing number of experienced middle-aged nurses is important in order to retain this cohort and attract newly-departed, but still qualified, nurses back into the profession (Buchan, 1999). Measures to retain nurses as the workforce ages could include more flexible working arrangements, higher salaries and an increase in the retirement age (Buchan, 1999). Nurses cited the following factors as influencing their decision to delay retirement: improved finances, reduced hours (if no effect on pension), reduced stress, feeling valued for their contribution, time out and flexibility of work (RCN, 2004a). Experienced nurses choose to work in areas with more choice, higher levels of part-time work and more control over working hours.

Between 1999 and 2003, only 3000 to 4500 nurses and midwives have returned to nursing from other sectors. It is not certain how many 'returners' stay on after the initial retraining, nor how many leave early or late (RCN, 2004a).

The nursing profession needs to be made more attractive to overseas students so that they remain in the UK (Finlayson *et al.*, 2002b). At present, many training places are filled by overseas students who are less likely to remain in the UK to work (Finlayson *et al.*, 2002b). There is a question as to why the social work degree has attracted more people, while the nursing degree has not (General Social Care Council, 2004).

At the end of 2004, the Department of Health published a revised code of practice for the recruitment of overseas healthcare professionals. From December 2005, employers will no longer be able to recruit actively from developing countries. For

---

[7] Relative earnings for nurses have decreased in relation to the non-manual jobs over the last 30 years. London and the South East are hard hit because nurses cannot afford to live there on present earnings (Batata, 2004).

[8] The employment opportunities have increased for women.

the first time, the code will be applied to the independent health sector too. People from developing countries will, however, still be able to apply directly for jobs in the UK (Cottell, 2005).

Nurses often start their careers within the NHS and although they may leave the NHS later, they may still be working as nurses. The number of UK-trained nurses leaving the country to work abroad has also increased. More than 8000 nurses left the UK between 2000/01 and 2002 (BBC News, 2004). Almost half of the nurses who leave the NHS remain in caring occupations, for example social or child care thereby contributing to the care workforce (Gage et al., 2001). Approximately 25% of RCN members report that they work outside the NHS (RCN, 2004a).

Policy responses to the shortage of nurses address: pay and work conditions, the development of careers,[9] nurse education (RCN, 2001; 2004b) and role expansion. For nurses and other professionals, training is provided with public funds, yet they often do not remain within the public sector after training. Policymakers need to consider whether a levy would prevent such behaviour.

There is a global shortage of qualified nurses, particularly in developed countries. This has led to increasing competition for recruitment and retention. In North America and Australia, nursing salaries have increased as a result of such global trends. The workforce strategy *Agenda for Change* proposes that nurses and all other health sector workers are paid on an equitable and transparent basis in the UK (DH, 2004a). In addition to improvements in basic salary, terms and conditions of employment – family-friendly policies, more flexible approaches to time off duty and holidays and support for continuing professional development – are aspects of employers' commitment to growing and sustaining the nursing workforce.

The medical workforce

Medicine is experiencing significant change in its role and working methods. An emphasis on self-care may shift the doctor role from 'heroic interventionist' to supporter and maintainer of self-care. The medical workforce is changing too. The UK has fewer doctors per capita than the rest of Europe. Doctors are ageing and retiring (early) and certain cohorts are not being replaced. Wanless predicts that the rise in primary care activity will require a doubling of GPs in the future and that overall there will be a shortage of 25 000 doctors by 2022 (Wanless, 2002).

The proportion of GPs intending to leave direct patient care in England within five years rose from 14% in 1998 to 22% in 2001. The main reasons given were increased age, job dissatisfaction, having no children under 18 years of age and ethnic minority status (Sibbald et al., 2003). The main causes for men leaving practice were related to age, their own ill health or death while for women they were related to family, emigration or taking on a non-medical post (BMA, 2004b). A Scottish survey indicates that of GPs in Scotland now aged 55 and above, at least 71% plan to retire at or before the age of 60, with excessive workload being cited as the main reason (Chambers et al., 2004).

---

[9] Such as specialist, advanced and consultant nursing roles that are emerging as part of an overall strategy to develop more effective careers for nurses. Research has demonstrated that nurses stay longer in clinical practice when they have more control of their work and can operate more autonomously (Aiken et al., 2002).

Most junior doctors who leave the UK to work abroad want a different lifestyle but to remain in medicine. A smaller group cite their experience of working as a doctor in the UK as the reason for leaving (Moss *et al.*, 2004). Extreme stress plays a serious role in increasing the turnover of doctors. It is highest in inner cities, where costs of living are typically at a maximum and lifestyle factors may encourage doctors to relocate (Peter *et al.*, 2004). Doctor shortages and high turnover impact negatively on patient care, healthcare costs and workplace morale.

In addition to pressure created by the European Working Time Directive,[10] two European Court rulings have had an impact on the definitions of work and rest time (Sheldon, 2004). Hours asleep, while on duty and if not busy, are counted as work (Watson, 2004) and doctors must have immediate compensatory rest (Moore, 2004). More doctors may be needed in the UK as a consequence of the ruling and job responsibilities may need to be restructured. In certain hospitals, a 24-hour matron service has been initiated to replace some of the aspects junior doctors cover (Carr-Hill *et al.*, 2003). Nurses are taking over many of the responsibilities that were formally the preserve of the doctor. The nurse is now often the first port of call for patients in primary care[11] and the co-ordinator of clinical care in secondary care[12] (Davies, 2003).

Shortfalls in doctor numbers could be addressed by expanding medical training to admit higher numbers of students, reforming the organisation of medical practices to use doctors' time more efficiently, taking steps to prevent or delay early retirement, retaining doctors through financial incentives and recruiting from abroad.

Figures from the Higher Education Funding Council for England show that 6030 students enrolled in medicine in 2003; 60% more than in 1997 (BBC, 2004c).[13] Increasing student numbers is a long-term solution, since it takes five years to complete a degree, and a further six to ten years to move to a more senior position. Furthermore, over 50% of medical graduates are now women (Royal College of Physicians, 2004; Skills for Health 2003).[14] By 2012, women doctors are predicted to outnumber men (Roberts, 2005). Since women more frequently express the desire for career breaks and part-time work arrangements, this will have significant implications for the future organisation of general practice and hospital working arrangements.[15] As a consequence, the traditional GP partnership may need to be reformed to reflect the demands of female doctors, particularly when considering

---

[10] Doctors are not meant to work more than 13 hours in any 24-hour period and are to take an 11-hour break before and after each such shift.

[11] Examples of new roles in primary care are prescription, screening, health promotion, and management of chronic disease.

[12] Examples of new roles in secondary care are minor injury services, cardiology day care, nurse endoscopists and night nurse practitioner.

[13] This increase is largely a result of the shift in funding of nursing courses to the higher education sector. However, there was also a substantial rise in enrolments in pharmacy, audiology, ophthalmics and medical technology.

[14] There is a continuing debate as to whether and how to attract men back into medical school (Ferriman, 2002). At present, only a quarter of all UK medical students are white male (Goldacre *et al.*, 2004).

[15] Up to 75% of female trainees said they planned to work part-time in the future. There is anecdotal evidence that men are expressing more interest in part-time work (Royal College of Physicians, 2004).

flexible work-time arrangements, work–life balance and childcare facilities (DH and NHS Alliance, 2004). Women also seem more interested in the 'softer' specialties (lower paid, less technical and more patient-focused)[16] (Akbar, 2004; Laurance, 2004a,b). This could result in more severe shortages in some areas, irrespective of patient demand and need (Harrison and Dixon, 2000).

In order to use doctors' time more efficiently, nurses may take over some of the current responsibilities of doctors. This would leave doctors to focus solely on work for which they alone are qualified (Horrocks *et al.*, 2002). It makes more sense in economic and managerial terms if patients are seen by nurses,[17] although the extended role of nurses has been slow to develop (Laurent, 2004). Consideration needs to be given to ensure that this solution does not merely shift the problem of shortages on to nurses.

Improving the quality of doctors' working lives could help improve retention (Pearson *et al.*, 2004; Sibbald *et al.*, 2003). The government has introduced financial incentives to encourage hospital doctors to enter general practice and to dissuade GPs from retiring early. To attract new graduates, 'golden hellos' have been introduced (DH and NHS Alliance, 2004). GPs have commented that a retention scheme needs to be flexible and well remunerated (Chambers *et al.*, 2004). The GP contract, between a Primary Care Trust (PCT) and a practice rather than an individual doctor, is seen as a measure to improve the GP's work situation by moving towards part-time or 'portfolio' GPs. It enables GPs to control their workload and it has been suggested that GPs can earn up to one-third more (Stevens, 2004). The contract has not been in place for long enough to know how income will change – it is likely that better-organised practices may earn more. Non-medical staff may be able to take over some jobs, and practices will become larger with sub-specialisation[18] (Healthcare Commission, 2004). In the future, general practitioners with special interest, GPwSIs, are likely to be more common (DH, 1997).

At present, overseas-trained doctors are filling gaps in supply. The accession of ten new member states to the EU means that thousands more doctors are eligible to work in the UK (BMA, 2004a). A draft directive of the mutual recognition of professional qualifications will aim to ensure patient safety and high standards of medical training (BMA, 2004a). In 2003, 5% of all doctors employed by the NHS in the UK had primary medical qualifications from the EEA/EU, and 24% had qualifications from non-EEA/EU countries (DH, 2004b). Of general medical

---

[16] Currently only 4% of women are consultant surgeons (Roberts, 2005).

[17] However, in its extreme, this delegation of work could mean that the doctor would only see a patient when a nurse or nurse practitioner was unable to handle a case (Charles-Jones *et al.*, 2003). That could pose a problem because sometimes the seemingly trivial problems are symptoms of something more serious, which only a doctor can diagnose and then this hierarchical delegation of resources becomes a problem. On the other hand, patients think that nurses are better communicators and might view this as an improvement in the patient-clinician relationship. Nurses who substitute for doctors spend more time with patients (Wanless, 2002).

[18] The family doctor and long-term relationship with the individual will disappear. The patient may be treated at the registered practice, another practice, by staff employed by the PCTs, or a community pharmacist.

practitioners,[19] 15% had qualifications from non-EEA/EU countries and 5% had qualifications from EEA/EU countries (Buchan, 1999). An informal study by the BMA shows that only 150 refugee doctors practise in the UK. A further 123 have qualifications to work but do not have jobs (BMA, 2004d).[20] Asylum seekers or refugees who are doctors with proper qualifications and experience should be allowed to practise once these qualifications have been assessed. In future we can expect a rise in doctors with non-British qualifications. Thought needs to be given to controlling or facilitating rising overseas recruitment and recognising its limitations.

Transforming care: shifting roles and professional boundaries

Although there is a constant shift between primary and secondary care, more conditions are now being managed by primary care (Skills for Health, 2003). The erosion of boundaries between professional groups, between professionals and informal carers, and between forms of care (such as social and healthcare) makes definitional distinctions difficult to uphold (Forbat and Henderson, 2003). While there are demands for professional groups to be flexible and change the way they train and work in the interests of patient-centred care, there is also a desire to preserve the highly valued professional status, practices, training and ethos typical of the health professional (Sausman, 2003). Any restructuring of the healthcare system would need to balance these tensions or manage them.

Many of the problems in healthcare services result from failure to work effectively across organisations and professional boundaries (Carr-Hill *et al.*, 2003). Some argue that this is due to doctors receiving different training from the rest of the health professions (Carr-Hill *et al.*, 2003). There is a need for training to work as a team and the leaning towards a non-hierarchical team structure will require different skills as well as attitudes (Skills for Health, 2003). Primary care services may need to be provided 24 hours a day, seven days a week and will affect working patterns (Skills for Health, 2003).

Level of qualification and quality of care do not always correlate. Patients have been shown to be more satisfied with nurse practitioners' than doctors' care because nurse practitioners have longer consultation times and make more investigations (Hewitt *et al.*, 2003). Midwifery care too has been rated by patients as comparable and sometimes better than care provided by obstetricians and other doctors (Hewitt *et al.*, 2003). Nurse practitioners are typically able to perform and manage simple procedures as well as doctors in primary and secondary care (Hewitt *et al.*, 2003). Their hours are cheaper although the cost savings implied may be outweighed by the fact that nurse practitioners take longer to do a given number of procedures. While there is some evidence that complicated care for serious cases is better

---

[19] This includes GMS Unrestricted Principals, PMS Contracted GPs, PMS Salaried GPs, Restricted Principals, Assistants, GP Registrars, Salaried Doctors (Para. 52 SFA), PMS Other and GP Retainers.
[20] Of the 951 doctors registered on the BMA/Refugee Council refugee doctors' database, 53 are working for the NHS, and some 450 are in various stages of qualifying.

performed by specialists,[21] (Hewitt *et al.*, 2003) certain tasks involved in treating common chronic diseases can be just as effectively performed by someone less qualified (Starfield, 2003).[22]

At present, nurses (and doctors) spend 25% of their time dealing with information rather than with patients (NPfIT, 2000). If some of that time can be released from paperwork by deploying healthcare assistants, ward clerks and housekeepers, it could make a difference, although research has not yet investigated the effectiveness of healthcare assistants or housekeepers within a caring team (Carr-Hill *et al.*, 2003). ICT may reduce time spent on administration and so alleviate some shortages.

The Health and Social Care Act (2001) authorised new prescribing powers for nurses and pharmacists. This shift from the former separation between prescribing and dispensing for pharmacists will have an impact on the way patients engage with their local GPs, nurses and pharmacists in the future. Whether it will lead to an increase in the number of prescriptions sold over the counter remains to be seen (Shannon, 2004).

Health and social care

Although integrating healthcare and social care might enhance care and focus on the patient, evidence is not conclusive that an integrated system is favourable to the current dual system (Hudson, 2002; Kendall and Harker, 2002; Rummery and Coleman, 2003), nor would integration be straightforward. In England, local authorities responsible for social care and the NHS have different planning timescales, accountability, funding and management structures (Baggott, 1998). There are also differences in professional orientation (medicine versus social models of health and wellbeing), professional status, knowledge base ('hard' sciences versus 'soft'), applications of technology ('high' and 'esteemed' versus 'low' and 'not esteemed'), action ('direct' versus 'vague', for example 'surgery' versus 'conversation'), legitimacy and power ('real' life-and-death needs versus 'disputed' needs) (Hudson, 2002). Issues such as who prioritises care-giving and who ensures that people do not fall through a gap between care structures need to be given consideration. Older people in particular must not be overlooked or cared for inappropriately on either side of the boundary (Lewis, 2001). Before considering integrated care, the care approach of Northern Ireland should be evaluated[23] since there may be a mismatch between policy pointed to integrated care and the reality of integrated care.

The debate between healthcare, free at the point of delivery, and social care services, which are largely means-tested, continues (Rummery and Coleman,

---

[21] Specialists provide better palliative care, A&E care, cardiac care, and care in more rare and serious situations. However, for musculoskeletal diseases there is little evidence that specialist doctors provide better care than generalists. In the case of Parkinson's disease, a nurse specialist in a hospital setting can improve outcomes and reduce costs. A community nurse can do the same with diabetes (Hewitt *et al.*, 2003).

[22] Specific tasks within cancer care are rectal surgery and sigmoidoscopies.

[23] In Northern Ireland, health and social services are commissioned and delivered by joint health and social service boards (Skills for Health, 2003).

2003). The Royal Commission on the Funding of Long Term Care recommended that nursing and personal care be provided free at the point of delivery on the basis of assessed need. This has led to different policy directions in England and Scotland. While personal care[24] and nursing care are free in Scotland, in England personal care is means-tested.

Conclusions

This discussion throws up a host of general questions for healthcare policy. As society's values shift from social obligations to greater individualism and increased levels of participation in the economy, is it realistic to expect informal carers to step into the breach associated with an ageing population? In the area of formal or paid care, can increasing recruitment objectives be satisfied while rates of pay are so low? Should alternative and complementary care be regulated to ensure a standard of quality? Is the impact of self-care strategies on the additional amount of information, advice and support required for those with long-term medical conditions fully understood? Should GPs use alternative and complementary therapies if there is so little evidence of their effectiveness? Is the current flow into the NHS of new nurses and doctors sustainable? In particular, can we continue to rely on overseas recruitment to address domestic skills shortages? Should recruitment agencies be regulated? How should the flow of nurses and doctors into the country be monitored (Buchan and Sochalski, 2004)? How are the boundaries between self-care, unpaid, informal, paid and professional care managed? And what skills, knowledge and attributes do carers need to operate safely and effectively in each of these areas? How can local strategies for recruitment correspond to local needs?

One of the main challenges facing society as the demand for care grows will be the current and future shortage of health and social care staff to meet this demand. The issues of an ageing population and the emergence of more complex chronic diseases and long-term mental health conditions will require policymakers and professionals to think differently about care, how we deliver it and, perhaps most importantly, how we improve it.

Care is not a clearly defined concept within the health and social policy arena. This leads to blurring of boundaries between who cares (the person, family or friends, a health or social care worker or a professional), whether they are paid for it (when informal, unpaid care become paid, formal care) and where care is received (in the patient's home or in an institution). With this lack of conceptual clarity comes the challenge of identifying how we are to evaluate effective caring interventions and who is best placed to provide that care.

Whatever the current definition, trends indicate that in the future there will be an insufficient number of carers to cope with people requiring care, whether that be from informal carers, support workers or professionals. Workforce strategies need to address issues of remuneration, intervention recruitment, interagency working and training and development.

---

[24] Personal care includes bathing, feeding and dressing.

Policy recommendations

- How self-care is taught, learned, maintained and sustained is essential to the future.
- The effects of incentives for self-care, educational programmes and training in IT (since access to information is the foundation of self-care) need to be investigated, as does the identification of triggers that identify when an individual is no longer able to self-care effectively.
- Incentives for informal carers, how they can be best supported financially and emotionally and how they can share their expertise need to be considered, because although there is some support for informal carers, caring can be financially impoverishing and stressful.
- Social care must be recognised as integral to health, healthcare and wellbeing.
- While many studies list a wide variety of local NHS policies and interventions in response to staff shortages, there needs to be evaluation of the effectiveness of these interventions.
- Research is required into the competitiveness of NHS pay and conditions compared to other areas of employment and into the number of healthcare workers needed before effective policy can be put in place.
- Following changes in employment contracts and an increase in investment with implications for pay and pensions in the future, the effect of pay and other terms and conditions of doctors and nurses on recruitment and retention needs to be monitored. Research to evaluate their cost and clinical effectiveness on patient care is also required.
- Projections about the required size and nature of the professional workforce cannot be done in isolation. The whole complex relationship between self-care, informal and paid care needs to be factored into professional workforce equations.
- With frequent organisational changes, the impact of changing clinical roles needs to be monitored. For example, delegating tasks to nurses and nurse practitioners frees up time for doctors but more research has to be conducted into how this 'freed' time is spent.
- As the main reason for women doctors leaving the profession is their family, thought needs to go into accommodating this obligation, with development of appropriate family-friendly employment policies.
- The pros and cons of international recruitment of doctors and nurses, and whether it is a sustainable option for meeting future workforce needs must be explored and policy developed in a global context.

References

Aiken LH, Clarke SP, Sloane DM, Sochalski J and Silber JH (2002) Hospital nurse staffing and patient mortality, nurse burnout and job dissatisfaction. *Journal of American Medical Administration*. **288**(16): 1987–93.

Akbar A (2004) Warning over women's role in medicine backed by male peers. *The Independent*. 3.8.04.

Baggott R (1998) Care in the community. In: *Health and Healthcare in Britain*. Macmillan Press, London, pp. 228–47.

Batata A (2004) *Why might nurses choose not to work for the NHS?* Strategic Issues in Healthcare Management (SICHM), St Andrews.

BBC (2004a) Care services costs set to rise. http://news.bbc.co.uk/1/hi/england/tyne/3888941.stm. Accessed: 27 July 2004.

BBC (2004b) 'Golden hello' for social workers. http://news.bbc.co.uk/1/hi/england/lincolnshire/3576957.stm. Accessed: 4 August 2004.

BBC (2004c) Record number of trainee doctors. http://news.bbc.co.uk/1/hi/health/3545991.stm. Accessed: 2 June 2004.

BBC (2004d) Social work recruitment 'success'. http://news.bbc.co.uk/1/hi/scotland/3631157.stm. Accessed: 4 August 2004.

BBC News (2004) Foreign nurse drive unsustainable. http://news.bbc.co.uk/1/hi/health/3703093.stm. Accessed: 15 May 2004.

BMA (2004a) *Annual Report of Council 2003–2004*. British Medical Association, London.

BMA (2004b) *Career Barriers in Medicine: doctors' experience*. British Medical Association, London.

BMA (2004c) *Health Policy Debate – May 2004*. British Medical Association, London.

BMA (2004d) Refugee doctors: a BMA briefing paper. http://www.bma.org.uk/ap.nsf/Content/RefugeeDocsBriefingPaper. Accessed: 2 June 2005.

Buchan J (1999) The 'greying' of the United Kingdom nursing workforce: implications for employment policy and practice. *Journal of Advanced Nursing*. **30**(4): 818–26.

Buchan J and Sochalski J (2004) The migration of nurses: trends and policies. *Bulletin of the World Health Organization*. **82**(8): 587–94.

Carers UK (2002) *Without Us ...? Calculating the value of carers' support*. Carers UK, London.

Carmichael F and Charles S (1998) The labour market cost of community care. *Journal of Health Economics*. **17**(6): 747–65.

Carr-Hill R, Currie L and Dixon P (2003) *Scoping Exercise. Skillmix in Secondary Care. SDO 'Scoping' Exercise*. Centre for Health Economics, University of York, York.

Chambers M, Colthart I and McKinstry B (2004) Scottish general practitioners willingness to take part in a post-retirement retention scheme: questionnaire survey. *British Medical Journal*. **328**: 329.

Charles-Jones H, Latimer J and May C (2003) Transforming general practice: the redistribution of medical work in primary care. *Sociology of Health & Illness*. **25**(1): 71–92.

Christakis NA (2004) Social networks and collateral health effects. *British Medical Journal*. **329**: 184–5.

Cottell C (2005) Is this the way to treat nurses who want a job? *The Guardian*. 5.2.05.

CPPIH (2004) Commission for Patient and Public Iinvolvement in Health website. http://www.cppih.org/index.html. Accessed: 4 October 2004.

Davies C (2003) Introduction: a new workforce in the making? In: C Davies (ed.) *The Future Health Workforce*. Palgrave Macmillan, Basingstoke, pp. 1–13.

DH (1997) *The NHS Plan: a first class service*. Department of Health, London.

DH (2000) *The NHS Plan: a Plan for investment, a plan for reform. Cmnd 4818–I*. Department of Health, London.

DH (2001) *Learning from Bristol. The report of the public inquiry into children's heart surgery at the Bristol Royal Infirmary 1984–1995*. Department of Health, London.

DH (2003) *Domiciliary Care: national minimum standards regulations*. Department of Health, London.

DH (2004a) *Agenda for Change*. Department of Health, London.

DH (2004b) All NHS doctors by country of primary medical qualification. Personal communication. Email to: LR Chang.

DH (2005a) *Independence, Well-being and Choice: our vision for the future of social care for adults in England: Social Care Green Paper. Cmnd 6499*. Department of Health, London.

DH (2005b) *Self Care – A Real Choice: self care support – a practical option*. Department of Health, London.

DH and NHS Alliance (2004) *A GP Recruitment and Retention Primer. Initiatives to improve recruitment and retention of GPs. For PCTs, Deaneries, WDCs and individual practices*. Department of Health, NHS Alliance, London.

Eborall C and Garmeson K (2001) *Desk Research on Recruitment and Retention in Social Care and Social Work*. Department of Health, London.

EOC (2004) *The Care Workforce*. Equal Opportunities Commission, London.

Ferriman A (2002) Men should be encouraged to apply to medical school. *British Medical Journal*. **325**: 66.

Finlayson B, Dixon J, Meadows S and Blair G (2002a) Mind the gap: the extent of the NHS nursing shortage. *British Medical Journal*. **325**: 538–41.

Finlayson B, Dixon J, Meadows S and Blair G (2002b) Mind the gap: the policy response to the NHS nursing shortage. *British Medical Journal*. **325**: 541–4.

Forbat L and Henderson J (2003) The professionalisation of informal carers? In: C Davies (ed.) *The Future Health Workforce*. Palgrave Macmillan, Basingstoke, pp. 49–67.

Gage H, Pope R and Lake F (2001) Keeping nurses nursing: a quantitative analysis. *Nursing Times*. **97**: 35–7.

General Social Care Council (2003) First wave organisations for English Social Care Register announced. http://www.gscc.org.uk/news_story.asp?newsID=70. Accessed: 15 March 2005.

General Social Care Council (2004) Record numbers enthusiastically enter social work training. http://www.gscc.org.uk/news_story.asp?newsID=117. Accessed: 6 March 2005.

Goldacre M, Davidson JM and Lambert TW (2004) Country of training and ethnic origin of UK doctors: database and survey studies. *British Medical Journal*. **329**: 597–600.

The Guardian (2004) Social care staff: the issue explained. *The Guardian*. 6.1.04.

Guberman N, Nicholas E, Nolan M, Rembicki,D, Lundh U and Keefe J (2003) Impacts on practitioners of using research-based assessment tools: experiences from the UK, Canada and Sweden with insights from Australia. *Health and Social Care in the Community*. 11(4): 345–55.

Harrison A and Dixon J (2000) *The NHS: facing the future*. King's Fund, London.

Healthcare Commission (2004) *State of Healthcare Report*. Healthcare Commission, London.

Henwood M (2001) *Future Imperfect: report of the King's Fund care and support inquiry*. King's Fund, London.

Hewitt C, Lankshear A, Maynard A, Sheldon T and Smith K (2003) *Health Service Workforce and Health Outcomes. A Scoping Study. Final Report*. Department of Health Sciences, University of York, York.

Horrocks S, Anderson E and Salisbury C (2002) Systematic review of whether nurse practitioners working in primary care can provide equivalent care to doctors. *British Medical Journal*. **324**: 819–23.

Hudson B (2002) Integrated Care and Structural Change in England: the case of care trust. *Policy Studies*. **23**(2): 77–95.

Hutt R and Buchan J (2005) *Trends in London NHS Workforce: an updated analysis of key data*. King's Fund, London.

Iles A (2003) Forty per cent of carers have illness or disability. *British Medical Journal*. **327**: 832.

Johnson A (2004) *Pathways to work: enabling rehabilitation*. http://www.dwp.gov.uk/aboutus/2004/18_10_04_prrsm.asp. Accessed: 1 April 2005.

Kendall L (2001) *The Future Patient*. Institute for Public Policy Research, London.

Kendall L and Harker L (2002) *From Welfare to Wellbeing: the future of social care*. Institute for Public Policy Research, London.

King's Fund (2005) Wanless Social Care Review. http://www.kingsfund.org.uk/healthpolicy/wanless.html. Accessed: 1 March 2005.

Laurance J (2004a) The medical timebomb: 'too many women doctors'. *The Independent*. 2.8.04.

Laurance J (2004b) President of Royal College speaks out on pressures for women in medicine. *The Independent*. 2.8.04.

Laurent C (2004) Where do they come in? *Health Service Journal*. **114**: 34.

Lewis J (2001) Older people and the health-social care boundary in the UK: half a century of hidden policy conflict. *Social Policy and Administration*. **35**(4): 343–59.

Marshall H (2004) NHS spends on agency staff as vacancies rise. *The Scotsman*. 13.8.04.

McLean S and Mason JK (2003) The law and the elderly. In: *Legal and Ethical Aspects of Healthcare*. Greenwich Medical Media, London, pp. 225–35.

MENCAP (2005) Benefit changes aim to get people working. http://www.mencap.org.uk/html/news/story.asp?Story=338. Accessed: 1 April 2005.

Moore A (2004) They've already had five years' extra dispensation so you'd think they'd have got it right. *Health Service Journal*. **114**: 10.

Moss P, Lambert T, Goldacre M and Lee P (2004) Reasons for considering leaving UK medicine: questionnaire study of junior doctors' comments. *British Medical Journal*. **329**: 1263–5.

NHS (2004) Expert patients programme. http://www.expertpatients.nhs.uk/index.shtml. Accessed: 3 October 2004.

NPfIT (2000) *NPfIT vision to support the NHS modernisation programme*. http://www.npfit.nhs.uk/worldview/comment2/. Accessed: 5 March 2005.

Pearson R, Reilly P and Robinson D (2004) Recruiting and developing an effective workforce in the NHS. *Journal of Health Service Research Policy*. **9**(1): 17–23.

Peter EH, Macfarlane AV and O'Brien-Pallas LL (2004) Analysis of the moral habitability of the nursing work environment. *Journal of Advanced Nursing*. **47**(4): 356–64.

Princess Royal Trust for Carers (2004) Shocking new figures on number of kids caring. http://www.carers.org/news/press-releases-detail.asp?dsid=2238. Accessed: 1 September 2004.

PSSRU (2003a) *Future Demand for Long-Term Care 2001 to 2031*. Personal Social Services Research Unit, Canterbury.

PSSRU (2003b) *Home care workers: careers, commitments and motivations*. Personal Social Services Research Unit, Canterbury.

Rankin J (2004) *Developments and trends in mental health policy*. Institute for Public Policy Research, London.

RCN (2001) *Higher Education Project: charting the challenge for nurse lecturers in higher education*. Royal College of Nursing, London.

RCN (2004a) *The Future Nurse: trends and predictions for the nurse workforce*. Royal College of Nursing, London.

RCN (2004b) *Quality Education for Quality Care: priorities and actions*. Royal College of Nursing, London.

Research Works (2001) *Perceptions of Social Work and Social Care: report of findings*. Department of Health, London.

Roberts J (2005) The feminisation of medicine. *British Medical Journal Careers*. **330**: 13–15.

Rogers J (2002) *Support Staff in Health and Social Care: an overview of current policy issues*. Institute of Current Policy Research, London.

Royal College of Physicians (2004) *Women and Medicine*. Royal College of Physicians, London.

Rummery K and Coleman A (2003) Primary health and social care services in the UK: progress toward partnership? *Social Science & Medicine.* **56**: 1773–82.

Sausman C (2003) The Future Health Workforce: an overview of trends. In: C Davies (ed.) *The Future Health Workforce.* Palgrave Macmillan, London, pp. 222–41.

Shannon C (2004) Over the counter revolution. *Health Service Journal.* **114**: 30.

Sheldon T (2004) Pressure mounts over European Working Time Directive. *British Medical Journal.* **328**: 911.

Sibbald B, Bojke C and Gravelle H (2003) National survey of job satisfaction and retirement intentions among general practitioners in England. *British Medical Journal.* **326**: 22–6.

Sibbald B, Shen J and McBride A (2004) Changing the skill-mix of the healthcare workforce. *Journal of Health Services Research & Policy.* **9**(1): 28–38.

Skills for Health (2003) *A Health Sector Workforce Market Assessment 2003.* Skills for Health, London.

Starfield B (2003) The relationship between primary care, income inequality, and mortality in US states 1980–1995. *Journal of the American Board of Family Practice.* **16**(5): 412–22.

Stevens S (2004) Reform strategies for the English NHS. *Health Affairs.* **23**(3): 37–44.

Wanless D (2002) *Securing our Future Health: taking a long-term view.* HM Treasury, London.

Wanless D (2004) *Securing Good Health for the Whole Population: final report.* HM Treasury, London.

Watson R (2004) EU proposes changes to working time directive. *British Medical Journal.* **329**: 761.

Chapter 6

What will be the burden of health?

Linda Rosenstrøm Chang, Domhnall MacAuley and Zoë Slote Morris

Disease[1] is dynamic: patterns of morbidity change, the socio-economic context varies and individual response is influenced by alterations in health policy and technology. The current burden of health and possible future developments across a spectrum of uncertainty are explored in this chapter.

The success of contemporary health systems and medical progress in preserving life is increasing the burden of health. Trends identified in Chapter 1 suggest that, as the population ages and lifestyles change, the burden of chronic disease and mental illness will become an increasing challenge. While the impact and burden of infectious disease is less predictable, as is the burden of bio-terrorism, in order for the state to protect health a policy response for each of these scenarios is required.

This chapter focuses on the social and service implications for disease trends, and considers some of the issues relevant to them. It offers a discussion of public health policy in the context of persistent socio-economic inequality, and current policy focus on transferring responsibility for health from the state to the individual.

Chronic disease

Chronic disease is difficult to define. Last (2001) defines it as a health-related state lasting a long time, while the US National Center for Health Statistics' definition describes a condition of three months' duration or longer. The DH has not published a definition but its use of the term usually includes diseases that are expected to last for a year or more (Parkes, 2004).

The DH has not calculated the overall number of deaths attributable to chronic disease, nor how much is spent on chronic disease treatment every year. Spending on the disease-focused National Service Frameworks (NSFs) was estimated to be £9.9 billion in 2002–03[2] (Parkes, 2004), and Murphy estimates that chronic disease accounts for 78% of all healthcare spending in the UK (Murphy, 2004).

The Royal College of Physicians estimates that more than a fifth of the population suffers from a chronic disease today (Locker, 2003). By 2025, this is likely to rise to around half the population (Pink and Prior, 2004). Up to 80% of all GP visits (180 million yearly) in the UK are related to chronic disease[3] (DH, 2004a) and the burden is growing as the population ages. The World Health Organization (WHO) estimates

---

[1] For a definition of disease, illness, sickness and health *see* Chapter 3.
[2] This only covers CHD, cancer, renal disease, mental health and diabetes.
[3] 86% of all the problems people bring to primary care in the NHS are managed entirely in primary care, only 14% are referred to specialists (Yuen, 2000).

a doubling of chronic disease in the over 65 cohort by 2030 (Batty, 2004). Coronary heart disease (CHD) and cancer, in particular, while shifting towards chronic or managed forms of disease, also remain principal causes of premature death. The NHS has recently published a strategy to improve care for people with chronic diseases (DH, 2005) but has not included a definition, a list of chronic diseases, or an evaluation of chronic disease management (Lewis and Dixon, 2004).

Coronary heart disease (CHD)

Whilst death rates from CHD have fallen since the late 1970s in the UK, morbidity does not seem to be falling and, in some age groups, may even be rising (Kelly and Stanner, 2003). Levels of intervention are increasing and this has implications for healthcare costs.

According to the British Heart Foundation, between 2001 and 2004 the number of statins being prescribed has more than doubled, as has the number of re-vascularisation procedures (British Heart Foundation, 2004a). CHD is estimated to be the most costly disease in the UK (British Heart Foundation, 2004a), with statins costing more than any other class of drug and direct treatment costing the UK's healthcare system around £1.75 billion (British Heart Foundation, 2004b). Although this is more than any other country in the EU, per capita the UK still has the highest level of mortality (Bloomfield, 2005).

The overall annual cost of heart disease in the UK is calculated to be over £7.5 billion because it includes 400 000 informal carers, estimated to contribute care worth nearly £2.5 billion (Bloomfield, 2005; British Heart Foundation, 2004a). This raises the estimated cost of CHD more than seven times since previously published figures focused on healthcare costs alone (British Heart Foundation, 2004a). In addition, the cost to the economy in terms of lost earnings associated with CHD is estimated to total £3 billion (British Heart Foundation, 2004a).

Cancer

Cancer is another growing burden, since it is an age-related condition and the population is ageing. At present one out of three people suffer from cancer in their lifetime (Wanless, 2002). By 2024 this figure could increase by 23% in Wales and Scotland, 21% in England and 19% in Northern Ireland totalling 100 000 new cases of cancer in the age group over 65 (BMJ, 2004). Survival rates for some cancers are improving and are likely to keep improving due to earlier detection and improved treatment (Boyle et al., 2003).

Although the economic burden of cancer has not yet been thoroughly researched, there is general acceptance that it will increase. This is not only because of the ageing population, but because the diagnosis and treatment of cancer are changing rapidly. There are moves towards more targeted (and therefore probably more expensive) treatments, for example, and these are likely to expand over the next 15 years (Bosanquet and Sikora, 2004; Foot, 2004).

The UK Office of Health Economics puts the total NHS expenditure on cancer services in 2000–01 at £2106 million, or 10.6% of all disease costs (Bosanquet and Sikora, 2004). This represents a spending increase of 52% since 1990–91, while total healthcare spending increased by 12%. It does not take into account the full effects of extra investment promised in the NHS Cancer Plan (Bosanquet and

Sikora, 2004; DH, 2000) although, despite a £2 million investment, a recent report states that the Plan is 'delivering poor value for money' (Sikora *et al.*, 2005).

Chronic disease is associated with huge costs due to disease management and the fact that people are increasingly living with a disease rather than dying from it. It is estimated that primary prevention alone will reduce cancer mortality rates by 20% by 2010 (NHS, 2003; Wanless, 2003), for example, and this will increase the number of people known to be living with cancer.

Life expectancy, morbidity and the burden of disease

Debate about the impact of increasing life expectancy and associated morbidity – and whether it is compressing[4] (Fries, 1980) or not (Crimmins, 2001; Doblhammer and Kytir, 2001; McCallum, 1999) – may have been superseded by two further issues.

The first is McCallum's (2001) belief that any notion of compressed morbidity must also capture what he calls co-morbidity or sub-morbidity.[5] Co-morbidity is now the norm and health services must be able to care for people suffering from more than one disease at a time (McCallum, 2001; Pink and Prior, 2004).

The second issue involves a shift in the burden of disease: while some diseases such as coronary heart conditions have declined, others – for example cancers, dementia, and HIV – are increasing.[6] A recent report on adolescent health from the British Medical Association (2003), for example, suggests that life expectancy could even fall, given the declining health status of young people associated with increasing levels of alcohol misuse and obesity (BMA, 2003; Fontaine *et al.*, 2003; House of Commons Health Committee, 2004). It seems unlikely, therefore, that the overall burden of disease will decline in the future, not least because new technologies allow 'new' diseases, such as attention deficiency hyperactivity disorder (ADHD), to be identified and managed (Wood, 1999).

Changing the organisation of care

Chronic disease management seems likely to involve a range of settings and actors. Since different care approaches, expertise and technology are required for chronic care as opposed to acute care, this will place great pressure on health services to reform (Lewis and Dixon, 2004; Rothman and Wagner, 2003). Prevention and treatment facilities and practices are likely to change, as are concentrations of physician specialties, medical technologies and costs. As the costs of care of various conditions increase, competition for resources between different specialties and between primary and secondary care will increase. Ultimately, rising trends in the incidence of chronic disease, and its shifting pattern, demand a reassessment of the practical limits of future healthcare. Rationing health services will continue to be inevitable due to the gap between supply and demand (King's Fund, 2001). If current rates of increase in health expenditures will not allow a general expansion of services overall, then should CHD facilities be replaced by cancer facilities? In

---

[4] Fries hypothesised that age at the time of initial disability will increase more than the gain in longevity, leading to fewer years of disability and a lower level of cumulative lifetime disability.
[5] Co- or sub-morbidity refers to a co-existent disease.
[6] Increasing cancer rates may be due to earlier detection.

terms of health workforce, should cardiologists replace psycho-geriatricians? Should resources be shifted from curative treatment to caring for chronic disease?

There are already tensions between which types of care should be supplied by the state and which paid for by the individual, questions about appropriate care – where it should be provided and who should care – and much debate about whether living longer but with disabilities is desirable. (For further discussion, *see* Chapter 3.) Another key question for policy concerns whether healthcare services can cope with the current and projected demand for qualified personnel associated with disease management. Chronic disease management is likely to be a primary care task. Already 86% of asthma, depression, hyperlipidaemia, hypertension, and gross obesity is already managed exclusively in primary care (Gray, 2004b). More patients cannot be moved to primary care without staff and resources increasing. This implies a shift in policy priority from acute to chronic care.

Managed care

A stronger focus on managed care may have implications for the way in which care is organised. Individualised care in general practice is the valued traditional model of care in the UK (Sweeney *et al.*, 1998). In certain circumstances, however, medical care by a multidisciplinary team may be more effective than individualised care. For example, multidisciplinary teams in specialist centres may provide the best quality diabetic care (Rothman and Wagner, 2003; Wagner, 2000). Achieving a rehabilitative environment takes time and carers need to be trained to provide personalised treatment (Morgan, 2003).

While most evaluated disease management programmes have been shown to improve the management of the chronic disease and health outcomes, there is no evidence regarding the components most important for improving quality of care, nor of a direct link between disease management and increased survival rates or quality of life improvement, nor of the cost effectiveness of such programmes. Further research and an evaluation of the costs and benefits of disease management should take place before it is introduced more broadly (Health Evidence Network, 2005).

Current trends in policy indicate a greater emphasis on self-care[7] in the future, partly as a response to a shortfall in doctors and rising costs of treatment. The well-informed management of asthma using well-defined clinical protocols is one domain in which self-care can take the strain off the health service (Asthma UK, 2004). There are many patients and conditions, however, which will continue to demand intensive and continuous professional intervention.

Preventing disease, protecting health

Another important dimension to reducing the burden of chronic disease relates to the prevention of ill health. Many chronic diseases, for example cancer and CHD, could be avoided by healthier lifestyles. A third of cancer deaths are linked to smoking (Health Education Authority, 1998) and similarly risk factors for CHD include smoking, diet, physical activity, obesity and alcohol (British Heart Foundation,

---

[7] *See* Chapter 5 for discussion on self-care.

2004a). For this reason, there is an increasing policy focus on persuading people to take more responsibility for their health (DH, 2004b; Wanless, 2002; 2004).

To date, primary care has undertaken much of this work (Bhopal, 2004) but whether it should continue to offer advice on diet, exercise and other lifestyle issues is contentious. There is some evidence of benefits in providing guidance on anti-smoking (Sausman, 2003) for example, but there is limited evidence for the effectiveness of primary care guidance overall (Ebrahim and Smith, 1997; Imperial Cancer Research Fund Oxcheck Study Group, 1995; Langham *et al.*, 1996; Riemsma *et al.*, 2003). This may be due to the prevention of disease being dependent on a complex range of variables beyond medicine, for example deprivation (Monaghan *et al.*, 2003).

While policy responses need to take account of a broader range of variables that impact on health, policymakers continue to place most emphasis on individuals and their behaviour (Beauchamp, 2001; Brocklehurst and Costello, 2003; Connely and Emmel, 2003; Holland, 2002; Kelly, 2004; Leowski, 1998). In a survey of public attitudes to public health policy by the King's Fund (Opinion Leader Research, 2004), 60% of those surveyed agreed that the most effective way of preventing disease would be to tackle poverty, while at the same time 89% stated that the individual is responsible for their own health.

Part of the reason why policymakers persistently fail to address the issue of the state's role regarding poverty may be because it impacts on uncomfortable assumptions and values about the role of the state and the role of its citizens. If the overall effect of medicine on health is small, however, then policy should address income inequality issues, rather than lifestyle projects.

The changing social contract and individualised care

Whether the state's role in health promotion should be to impart information to support individual choices or whether it should attempt to change actual behaviour by other means is debatable. The assumption is that whilst the citizen has a legitimate claim on the state to protect their health (Hill, 1996), the state has a similar claim in expecting individuals to guard their own health (de Grey, 2001).

To improve overall health, a measure of contingency might be introduced into the unconditional right to treatment, compelling individuals to modify their life-styles (Vallgarda, 2001), or even have an individualised health 'contract' (Halpern *et al.*, 2004). It is unlikely, though, that such a shift would absolve the state from providing care to those who have not fulfilled their part of the bargain.

To reduce the incidence of chronic disease, existing research tends to signal a need for policy to address structural causes of ill health, for example socio-economic inequality (Lalonde, 1974; Raphael, 2003),[8] as opposed to attempting to change behaviour through information.[9] Despite a lack of evidence relating to effectiveness of individual programmes, and considerable evidence of unsuccessful interventions

---

[8] The message of the Lalonde Report was that the great health issues of our time are rooted in human behaviour.
[9] Marmot (2004) discusses whether governments should address inequality though material inequality or through 'psychosocial disadvantage' (promoting participation of lower social classes to increase control over their environment).

(Ashton, 2004; Yach, 2004), a recent briefing paper from the Health Development Agency (HDA) cites a range of projects related to 'lifestyle' which appear to promote health (Kelly, 2004).

The need to place more policy focus on structural issues does not negate the need, or potential effectiveness of individualised care. It is only through detailed discussion with individuals that attitudes, fears, values and activities, which are relevant to their health, can be established (Donelly, 2004; Gray, 2004a). This raises questions of reconciling paternalism and autonomy, as discussed in Chapters 2 and 3. If the view is that the state is responsible for health promotion, lack of success in some areas may reflect the need for comprehensive policy designed to support health, the complexity of the issues, and human behaviour.

Since the benefits of health promotion are yielded in the future, there is little direct evidence of their effectiveness. The absence of 'good' data might suggest a greater need for innovative policy and there is nascent research indicating the ways in which this may develop (Halpern and Cockayne, 2004; Hillsdon *et al.*, 2004).

Prevention of chronic disease is not, therefore, simply a medical issue, but one with implications for industry, agriculture and the economy. In the context of globalisation, appropriate responses may lie beyond national governments,[10] for example, there has been an international push for governments to introduce national legislation on more accurate food labelling to help address obesity (Yach and Hawkes, 2004). The policymakers' crucial message has to be that medicine can help reduce problems associated with obesity but it cannot prevent them.

Mental health

Mental health is not easy to define (Lehtinen, 2003). One acceptable definition is: 'the state of successful performance of mental function, resulting in productive activities, fulfilling relationships with other people, and the ability to adapt to change and cope with adversity' (European Commission, 2004). It is important to remember that mental health influences overall health and mental illness can accompany, follow or precede physical disorder (Herrman, 2001).[11]

Defining 'mental illness' is still more problematic since it covers a wide spectrum ranging from universally-experienced worries and grief, to suicidal depression or complete loss of touch with everyday reality (Mental Health Foundation, 2004a). The World Health Organization has published a list of 11 mental and behavioural disorders, including, for example, 'organic' disorders – dementia and delirium, disorders due to psychoactive substance use, schizophrenia, schizotypal and delusional disorders, mood disorders, neurotic disorders and mental retardation (WHO, 2001a). There is, however, no universally-agreed division between what is considered 'normal' and what is considered a mental illness, and this is partly a

---

[10] For example, WHO is developing a strategy to address global obesity with dietary guidelines and prescriptions for physical activity and has encouraged food multinationals to change their products to include less salt and harmful fats.
[11] People suffering from mental illnesses tend to have shorter life expectancy than the general population (Trueland, 2004). A formal investigation, *Equal Treatment: closing the gap* launched in December 2004 by the Disability Rights Commission, will look into the health inequalities experienced by people suffering from learning disabilities and mental health problems.

reflection of differences between countries, cultures, social groups and social settings (Mental Health Foundation, 2004a).

The issue of defining mental health is not simply abstruse theory. Given the special legal status afforded to those with a mental illness, the definition can affect an individual profoundly. The 1983 Mental Health Act defines mental illness as the 'arrested or incomplete development of mind, psychopathic disorder and any other disorder or disability of mind.' More recently, in the Mental Health Bill (DH, 2004c), mental disorder is defined as 'An impairment of or a disturbance in the functioning of the mind or brain resulting from any disability or disorder of the mind or brain'. This wider definition extends to people with severe personality disorders. It captures a larger array of mentally ill categories and allows compulsory treatment on detention. The bill has been very controversial and a report by a parliamentary committee has just been published (Amos, 2004; Joint Committee on the Draft Mental Health Bill, 2004; 2005). Ministers have promised to re-examine the bill in light of the pre-legislative scrutiny by the expert parliamentary committee.

Definition of mental illness is also important to treatment. Although flawed, the categorisation of treatment and early detection of mental disorders has been shown to reduce the number of subsequent consultations, to shorten the duration of an episode, and to result in far less social impairment in the long term due to focus on the illness (Craig and Boardman, 1997). Early recognition and treatment, along with appropriate and sustained support for high-risk individuals and families, might avoid many problems.

The scale of the problem

WHO estimates that the burden of mental disease will increase from 12% of disease currently to 15% by 2020 and predicts an increase in incidence over time. Data from the Office of National Statistics (ONS), however, suggest that in the UK the prevalence of neurotic disorders (including mood disorders, for example depression) and psychotic disorders remained unchanged between 1993 and 2000 (WHO, 2003a). This may reflect a range of issues, including definitional, methodological and access, which makes assessing future demand for mental health services difficult. While one recent survey found that one in six adults experiences a mental health problem at some point, another major survey puts the figure at one in four[12] (Mental Health Foundation, 2004b). It is estimated that only half of the total number of mentally ill people are diagnosed (Cowper, 2004). About 6% of all consultations with GPs are for psychiatric disorders (Ashworth et al., 2003) and 20–30% relate to a mental health concern (Halliwell, 2004).

Mental illness is more common in disadvantaged social classes, people with long-term physical illness and unemployed, the homeless, elderly, bereaved and unmarried people (NHS Hertfordshire, 2004). Of pre-school children, 15% have mild mental health problems and approximately 7% have severe mental health problems. Six per cent of boys and 16% of girls aged 16–19 are thought to have some form of mental health problem and 8–11% of children and young people experience

---

[12] The one in six figure given by the ONS represents those people defined as having 'significant' mental health problems, whilst the one in four survey uses a wider definition of mental health problems.

anxiety to such an extent that it affects their ability to get on with their everyday lives (Mental Health Foundation, 2004a). Mental health problems suffered in childhood often continue into adulthood (DfES, 2004) and many adult disorders begin in adolescent years (Herrman, 2001).

Depressive disorders

Anxiety and depression, often occurring together, are the most prevalent mental disorders in the general population (Craig and Boardman, 1997). One woman in 15 and one man in 30 are affected by depression yearly. Approximately 44 adults per thousand are estimated to have an anxiety disorder (BBC News, 2004). Bunker has calculated that for every 100 individuals in society, there are 13–15 years of disability connected with depression (Bunker, 2001).

Depressive disorders are most common in those aged over 40 and are linked with other variables that are detrimental to health: social isolation, alcohol, drug abuse and smoking (Craig and Boardman, 1997; Herrman, 2001). Social ties and support can help to prevent or improve mental illness, even for diseases such as schizophrenia (IOM, 2003; Kawachi et al., 1997; Turner, 2004). Depression affects elderly people more than physical illnesses and is related to psychosocial factors, such as the death of a spouse, retirement, social isolation, and diminished income (Tanne, 2004). An increasing trend towards single-person households may increase levels of depression and other mental disorders in future.

The total cost of adult depression in England today is estimated at over £9 billion, of which £370 million represents direct treatment costs. There were 109.7 million working days lost and 2615 deaths due to depression in 2000. A decade ago, the estimated cost was £3.5 billion (Thomas, 2003).

Over the last five years, prescriptions of anti-depressant drugs have increased by 51% to 6.7 million items at a cost of £97 million (PPA, 2003). According to a Norwich Union healthcare poll, 72% of doctors prescribe more anti-depressant medication now than five years ago because of a lack of social care and counselling (BBC, 2004b). The rise in anti-depressant prescriptions could also be to do with better diagnosis and treatment (Morgan et al., 2004).

Although there is a lack of beds available to young people with mental health problems in the UK, the number of mental illnesses in young people is rising (White, 2004). According to WHO, depressive disorders are the fourth leading cause of disease and disability for children, and are expected to rise to second place by 2020 (WHO, 2003b). Suicide accounts for 20% of all deaths by young people and is connected to mental ill health (Mental Health Foundation, 2004a). Depression and low self-esteem are linked with other factors that are detrimental to young people's health such as smoking, binge drinking, eating disorders, drug misuse and unsafe sex (Herrman, 2001).

There is growing concern about the long-term side-effects of anti-depressant drugs, particularly when taken by children (Boseley, 2003; Jureidini et al., 2004), and a general lack of clinical data on the appropriateness of adult drugs for children (White, 2004). An increasing number of children are diagnosed with depression and, at the end of 2003, more than 50 000 children were prescribed anti-depressants (Timimi, 2004).

Stress

Stress is most often a natural and necessary reaction to a difficult situation. In a prolonged situation of stress, however, health and wellbeing can be affected, sometimes leading to depression, which is much more disabling (McEwan, 2004). Whilst the causal relationship between stress and disease has proven extremely difficult to establish, and there is no medical definition of stress, there does seem to be evidence that stress is a burden to the economy (McDaid, 2003). In 1992, the Confederation of British Industry and Percom suggested that, in a typical year, 80 million workdays are lost as a result of stress-related illness (CBI and DH, 1992). In 1996, half of all sickness from work was due to stress-related absences, costing an estimated £4 billion, with 182 000 cases of stress or depression either caused or made worse by work (Cooper and Cartwright, 1996). Self-perceived job insecurity has been shown to be associated with increased mental and physical ill health (Ferrie *et al.*, 2003), while being underemployed also contributes to poor mental health (Dooley, 2003). The issue of stress needs to be addressed by policy.

McEwan shows the connection between low socio-economic status and stress: poor people worry more about money, housing, employment and other day-to-day problems (McEwan, 2004). Since the UK has experienced an increase in income inequality over the last 20 years, this is likely to have adverse consequences for mental illness in the population (BMA, 2003). Some health outcomes appear to relate to social differences, rather than material differences (Marmot, 2004). The Whitehall study of civil servants, for example, found a higher prevalence of angina, diabetes, respiratory illness (only in men), poor self-rated-health and depression in individuals who rated themselves as having low social status,[13] as compared to those who saw themselves as having higher status (Singh-Manoux *et al.*, 2003). Stress is used to explain these differences (Wilkinson, 1996). Thus 'relative deprivation' – a lack of social relationships, social cohesion, or social capital, resulting from social inequalities – may be important to future mental health (Wilkinson, 1996).

Neurodegenerative disorders

One clear trend in mental illness is a rise in organic neurodegenerative disorders, associated with old age. One sixth of those aged 60–64 are relatively impaired in standard tests of memory and concentration, rising to one-quarter for those aged 70–74 (ONS, 2003a), and approximately 600 000 or 5% of the total population aged 65 years and above have dementia (DH, 2001). The risk of having dementia increases with age: one in 50 people aged 65–70 has a form of dementia, compared to one in five over the age of 80 (ILC, 2002). Half a million people suffer from Alzheimer's disease in the UK and this figure is expected to double within 20 years (ILC, 2002).

Research in improving or delaying Alzheimer's is underway but has yet to make any real impact (ILC, 2002). While drug therapy is offered to a smaller proportion of

---

[13] The subjective self-rated status is determined by occupational position, education, household income, satisfaction with standard of living, and feeling of financial security regarding the future.

Alzheimer patients in the UK (21%) than in other parts of Europe (Wilkinson *et al.*, 2004), the amount spent on dementia drugs has risen from £4.8 million in 2000 to over £22 million in 2003. The number of prescription items for dementia increased by nearly 80% between 2001/02 and 2002/03 (BBC, 2004c). In practice, this is likely to represent only a small part of potential healthcare costs.

Diagnosis of Alzheimer's takes an average of 32 months in the UK (BBC, 2004a), partly because only specialists can diagnose the disease and start treatment. This often requires a referral from the GP increasing the length of time before the patient can begin treatment (BBC, 2004a). Since treatment is most effective if started early (AD2000 Collaborative Group, 2004; Wilkinson *et al.*, 2004), expediting the process in the future will improve quality of life for sufferers and carers. It will also impact on healthcare costs.

Currently, Alzheimer's comes under social care, not medical care. In the UK, 62% of Alzheimer's patients are cared for by relatives (Wilkinson *et al.*, 2004) and up to 1.5 million people may be involved in caring for a relative or friend with a mental illness (Arksey, 2003). Practitioners suggest that, especially in the early stages, Alzheimer's should be managed in primary care. While rendering the categorisation of Alzheimer's under social care increasingly absurd, this would inevitably increase healthcare costs (Wilkinson *et al.*, 2004).

Mental health costs

Overall spending on mental health services has increased from 0.2% of GNP in 1954 to 0.3% by 1988. The allocation of resources for mental health is less than 12% of healthcare spending (Halliwell, 2004). Hospital care continues to absorb around 80% of NHS mental health expenditure, despite the overall number of NHS beds for the mentally ill dropping about 75% between 1954 and 2000 (Poole *et al.*, 2002). Taking pay and prices into account, the mental health budget in England is growing by 1.6%, compared with a 5% real-terms growth in the NHS budget as a whole (The Sainsbury Centre for Mental Health, 2003). Despite the fact that mental health is the government's third priority within the health service, mental health budgets are being squeezed because of staff shortages (high spending because of temporary staffing), an increase in prescribing costs, inherited debts that must be paid off and other NHS priorities (The Sainsbury Centre for Mental Health, 2003). Although an extra £1 billion was promised for the period 1997–2002, the impact, efficacy and exact amount allocated remains unclear (Rankin, 2004). The lack of transparency concerning resource allocation and actual spending needs to be addressed. Similarly, if the National Service Framework (NSF) for mental health is to be successfully implemented, a £3.1 billion increase would be needed by 2010–11 (Wanless, 2002). Overall, mental disorders are predicted to rise in an ageing population. An NHS primarily geared to treat physical conditions may be ill-equipped to deal with mental disorders on the scale necessary.[14] If mental health is the third priority within healthcare, more resources are needed to implement the NSF for mental health.

---

[14] In the UK, only 70 000 of the estimated seven million people who could benefit from psychotherapy actually do so (Cowper, 2004).

Who cares where?

The time spent in psychiatric care has decreased since the 1940s, when patients spent years in hospitals. Today, patients are generally discharged within one month (Morgan, 2003). The pressure on clinicians to discharge patients whenever feasible can lead to patients harming themselves or others, being discharged before they are ready and being released into the community when the community is not able to care for them (Kazarian *et al.*, 1997; McLean and Mason, 2003). In particular, shifting care outside the hospital places a heavy burden of care on informal carers.

The question of where it is preferable to treat mentally ill people is an ongoing debate. In 1994, the Audit Commission found that the favoured policy of treating the individual in the community was 'struggling' (Audit Commission, 1994). In 1998, then Health Secretary Frank Dobson declared that 'care in community has failed' (DH, 1998). This was an overstatement, but concern continues. The Royal College of Psychiatrists' study *The Living Project* investigates how people who were previously living in mental hospitals have fared in the community and will shed light on the quality of life of people with serious mental illness (The Royal College of Psychiatrists, 2005). The study will end in 2006. Community-based treatment is generally viewed as cheaper, although WHO has shown that treatments based in the community and hospitals are of equal costs, so a review of policy is needed (Health Evidence Network, 2004a). In general, the assumption has been that treatment in the community is preferable to that in a psychiatric ward or hospital because patients in mental institutions can lose touch with social reality if institutionalised over a long period.

Any future policy has to account for the fact that there is a shortfall in numbers of professionals and support staff caring for the mentally ill. Future studies should generate strategies for reducing excessive work burden and for improving recruitment and retention (Pajak *et al.*, 2003).

Mental health teams concentrate on mental illnesses and have little or no training in preventing and managing physical illness (Woodward and Ramsey, 2004). Training should be adjusted so that mental and physical diseases are linked rather than separated. Mental health teams may assume that patients are in contact with a GP or primary care services, but sometimes they are not (Woodward and Ramsey, 2004). This suggests a need for more integrated care. While improved outcomes of successful strategies for mental health are desirable, they are associated with increased healthcare costs (Health Evidence Network, 2004b).

Infectious disease

New infectious diseases and new variants of known infectious diseases are expected to emerge over the next 25 years (Singh, 2004). The spread of 35 new or newly-diagnosed infectious diseases over the past quarter century has been fuelled by the modern way of life (Singh, 2004). Main determinants of the spread of infectious diseases include nutrition, food and water safety, drug abuse, sexual behaviour, travel and access to quality healthcare (Wanless, 2003). Warfare also remains a condition particularly congenial to the spread of infectious diseases (Palmer *et al.*, 1999). In the near future, war is predicted to become a major contributor in the worldwide burden of disease (Lopez and Murray, 1998).

Sexually-transmitted diseases are on the rise. In the UK, HIV/AIDS currently presents the greatest single-infection threat, with infections in the UK increasing by 20% between 2001 and 2002 (Nicoll and Hamers, 2002; ONS, 2003b).[15] Many HIV-infected people originate from countries outside Europe. While statistics on HIV diagnosis are difficult to interpret – they rely on people seeking or being offered HIV testing and on accurate reporting – it costs between £500 000 and £1 million to prevent one adult from becoming infected (Nicoll and Hamers, 2002). Other sexually-transmitted diseases such as gonorrhoea and syphilis are also increasing in the UK,[16] with implications for fertility (BMA, 2003).

The incidence of tuberculosis (TB) infection in the UK is also on the rise due to homelessness, deprivation, an increase in drug-resistant strains and as a consequence of AIDS (Smith, 2001b). TB is nearly 100% curable and its spread can be controlled (Frieden, 2003). Although TB is cheap to treat, drug-resistant TB[17] is more than a hundred times more expensive because chemotherapy is required for treatment (WHO, 2004a). According to Frieden, mortality from TB could be reduced by over 80% in five years, and the prevalence reduced by more than 30%, by following policies on infectious diseases, ensuring effective clinical and public health management and coordinating efforts for its control from within and outside of the health sector. There is great uncertainty surrounding the threat posed by drug-resistant infections, but advances in biotechnology, molecular genomics and structure-based drug design may prevent regional outbreaks and global epidemics of potentially fatal and contagious drug-resistant diseases.

Most experts believe that future influenza pandemics are inevitable. They may be imminent and preparation should be made for them (Lazzari and Stohr, 2004; WHO, 2004b). Forecasting models of such threats predict that 20–50% of the population could fall ill (Communicable Disease Surveillance & Response (CSR), 2004) inflicting enormous economic damage worldwide (Lazzari and Stohr, 2004).[18] High projected costs of an influenza pandemic are estimated to come from morbidity, mortality and hospitalisation[19] (Balicer et al., 2004). The ability of the influenza virus to mutate, and occasionally take virulent and fatal forms, introduces both uncertainty and great danger (Louria, 2000).

If a new influenza subtype emerges in humans, mass vaccination would probably be the foundation of any control plan. Rates of success in generating vaccines against new subtypes is limited, despite more than 40 years' experience of administering inactivated vaccines for human influenza (Barclay, 2004) and so it is uncertain whether a vaccine could be prepared and manufactured in adequate

---

[15] The infection remains incurable. The potential to infect others is lifelong.

[16] Gonorrhoea increased by 102% from 1995–2000 in England and Wales, and was highest among older teenagers. Syphilis rose from 132 cases diagnosed in 1995, to 326 in 2000 (Nicoll and Hamers, 2002).

[17] Single- and multi-resistant TB exist – the former is resistant to one drug, the latter to more than one. Drug resistance is the result of inconsistent or partial treatment, patients stopping treatment because they feel better, because the incorrect treatment is prescribed, or because of unreliable drug supply (WHO, 2004b).

[18] In annual influenza outbreaks, 5–15% of the population is affected (WHO, 2003b).

[19] In the US, the cost has been estimated at over $100 billion.

numbers in time. According to WHO, drug companies should focus more on producing drugs for infections (Fleck, 2004).

A second concern is zoonotic infections (WHO Medicines and Policy Department (EDM), 2004). Recent influenza outbreaks in poultry are unprecedented in their scale, geographical spread and adverse economic effects among affected populations (Lazzari and Stohr, 2004). Because of high pathogenicity of avian influenzas in humans, there is growing concern that some of the influenza strains will cause a repeat of the Spanish flu[20] (Lazzari and Stohr, 2004). When dealing with zoonotic diseases, vaccinating poultry and developing poultry vaccines may be less problematic than generating human vaccines (Barclay, 2004).

At present, although few people in the UK die from infectious diseases[21] (Montgomery, 2003), they are expensive to treat (Balicer et al., 2004; DHPE, 2004; Nicoll and Hamers, 2002) and can cause serious morbidity and disability. Infectious diseases affect not only the victims, but also the people treating the disease. In dealing with SARS in Canada, Toronto healthcare staff suffered considerable emotional distress brought on not only by fear of infection but by isolation from friends and family (Nickell et al., 2004). This has wider implications for communicable disease control in public health in the future.

Preventing and responding to infectious diseases

Two major policy issues emerge. The first is a need for effective surveillance and monitoring. In a global context, the single most important measure for combating infection is the improvement of integrated surveillance and monitoring systems (Martens, 2002). The 2002 SARS outbreak demonstrated this need, as the infection travelled across national borders at the speed of long-distance aircraft. It also illustrated the need for public health institutions and disease prevention strategies geared to cope with infectious diseases. SARS highlighted the weaknesses in international co-operation on infectious disease control and provided the impetus for the creation of the European Centre for Disease Prevention and Control (ECDC)[22] (European Commission, 2003; The Wellcome Trust, 2004).

In order to limit the impact of infectious diseases in the future, plans need to be made on a European level now. The EU should take the lead in disease control by applying a long-term, systematic, strategic approach to crises (Smith, 2001a). The major weakness of the EU-wide collaboration of surveillance and monitoring is connected to the EU legislation which emphasises 'coordination of effort' rather than 'harmonisation of effort' (MacLehose et al., 2004). The EU needs to move beyond surveying to create a uniform approach to infectious disease.

---

[20] The last influenza pandemic in Europe, known as the Spanish flu, was in 1918–19. It killed more people than the First World War. Some experts believe that such pandemics recur periodically.

[21] This is contested by Wilson and Bhopal (1998) who claim that the international classification of diseases system hides the range of infectious diseases and conclude that the number of deaths attributed by infectious diseases was 6.7% between 1989 and 1993.

[22] THE ECDC is due to become operational in 2005 and will have four main tasks: 1 epidemiological surveillance and networking of laboratories; 2 early warning and response; 3 scientific opinions; 4 technical assistance and communication.

National responses to infectious disease control have also been inadequate. In England, the failure to respond effectively to the BSE and nvCJD crises illustrates organisational weakness, including lack of preparedness due to a confused responsibility for public health (Wanless, 2004). Monaghan *et al.* (2003) have highlighted some serious weaknesses in current public health measures in the UK, including a lack of clear responsibility. Failing to address structural issues is likely to weaken a response to any outbreak. One solution would be to establish a single UK-wide body dealing with public health (Monaghan, 2004).

At present governance structures and the distribution of ministerial and bureaucratic responsibility are fragmented (Monaghan *et al.,* 2003). Strengthening them and clearly defining the role of the Secretary of Health, for example, by extending the portfolio to matters of international relations, and clarifying the relationship between the Secretary of Health and the Home countries ministers responsible, would be a way forward.

Also, UK health policy operates in a global context and still needs to focus less on the domestic sphere (Collin and Lee, 2003). Globalisation changes the nature of health risks and the ways in which health systems must respond to them (Yach and Hawkes, 2004). It also provides opportunities to improve responses to disease and to access health findings and policies from across the globe. A cohesive and comprehensive globalisation and health research agenda addressing these new opportunities needs to be developed for the UK (Beaglehole and McMichael, 1999).

Health remains under-represented in policy discussions concerning global trade, investment, transport and other areas of relevance to global health (Beaglehole and Yach, 2003). The World Trade Organisation would like to ensure that the traditional services connected to health be offered by pharmaceutical companies, insurance companies and other service corporations (Price *et al.,* 1999).

Bio-terrorism

Bio-terrorism could be characterised as a deliberate attempt to use violence and intimidation in the pursuit of political aims through the use of biological or chemical agents. Biological agents include bacteria, viruses, toxins and rickettsia/coxiella (Parliamentary Office of Science and Technology, 2001). In the absence of a successful bio-terrorist attack, the primary policy issue relates to the diversion of funds given the perceived threat from bio-terrorism (IOM, 2003).

The spread of infectious diseases provides a glimpse into potential scenarios of bio-terrorism, with consequences for physical health, trade (losses because of public fear of eating particular foods), travel (a drop in tourism), civil liberties (the right to mobility restricted) (Gostin, 2001), security (increased measures to prevent a spread of the disease) and mental health (the stress of worry) (IOM, 2003). Emotional, behavioural and cognitive reactions range from insomnia, fear, anxiety and emotional vulnerability to increased alcohol consumption and smoking (IOM, 2003). Certain people suffering from the fear of attack may develop psychiatric illnesses, mimicking post-traumatic stress disorder (IOM, 2003). The perception of risk is a serious issue for the healthcare system, since anxiety itself has mental health consequences. Indeed, to a great extent, the fear of bio-terrorism represents a greater threat to health than the prospects of the threat itself (Furedi, 2002).[23] The likelihood of dying from food poisoning is much higher than being killed in a bio-terrorist attack.

Managing bio-terrorism

In terms of preparedness and prevention, vaccines can be given to either a high-risk segment of the population, or the whole of the population. They may be given as either a preventative measure or after exposure to a biological substance that causes disease (Parliamentary Office of Science and Technology, 2001). Prevention of death from biological terror agents can be highly problematic, however, and evidence is contradictory when using vaccines. Fearing the discomfort and side-effects of preventative vaccinations for anthrax, 500 American soldiers recently declined to be vaccinated after approximately 100 000 Persian Gulf War veterans became sick with a still unexplained syndrome which many suspect had to do with vaccines against chemical or biological weapons (Dyer, 2004; *The Economist,* 2003).[24]

WHO advises against using the smallpox vaccine for mass immunisation, in part because of the risk of adverse reactions (WHO, 2001b). Vaccination raises issues about the rights of the individual versus the common good, and policy needs to be clear about what can and should be expected of the individual. Fatalities connected to vaccinations are rising in the UK due to the greater prevalence of suppressed immune systems in the vaccinated population (WHO, 2004a). Statistically though, it is relatively safe to be vaccinated and only one to two people out of every million who receive the smallpox or flu vaccine will die from it (Buckley and Cohen, 2002; Greenberg, 1998).[25]

Few companies are prepared to produce the required smallpox vaccination (*The Economist,* 2003). The process of production can be high-risk in terms of product liability and costly in terms of pharmaceutical liability insurance. A portion of vaccines can have serious side-effects or be lethal. Governments will be the main buyers, making the industry very dependent on a small set of customers and there is uncertainty regarding maintenance of patents under certain circumstances. Furthermore, the cost of producing a new vaccine is immense (*The Economist,* 2003). Mass vaccination as a policy option for the future would involve addressing a range of issues.

The cost of preventing or preparing for a bio-terrorist attack is extremely high: the undertaking has been compared to the task of creating a missile-defence shield. US experts on bio-terrorism believe that around one hundred new diagnostics, vaccines and treatments are needed urgently. It is estimated that building bio-defences will cost $50 billion and take at least five to ten years (*The Economist,* 2004). The former General Secretary of the WHO, Gro Harlem Brundtland, has stated that better public health systems in general can prepare nations to detect and quickly contain incidents of bio-terrorism (Brundtland, 2004). A better understanding of the nature of the bio-terrorism threat, an early response plan, a means of dealing

---

[23] For the UK soldiers fighting in the first Gulf War, the threat of chemical warfare was the biggest fear (Unwin *et al.,* 1999).
[24] The side-effects were pounding headaches, nausea and memory loss.
[25] Smallpox is a virus that kills one in every three people it infects, and most survivors are disfigured.

with mass casualties and, when possible, an adequate stock of vaccines, even if the threat seems unlikely, and an adequate disease control system may be essential (*The Economist,* 2001). For population health, it is the fear, stress and anxiety connected to bio-terrorism which has major health consequences. A system to manage risk perception should be included in managing bio-terrorism.

Conclusions

This chapter considered the dynamic nature of disease, namely changing patterns of mortality and morbidity. It discussed potential threats to UK health in the future and some implications for policy. In selecting 'burdens' on which to focus, a range of challenges to health across a spectrum of certainty to uncertainty was explored.

Continued increases in chronic disease linked to an ageing population and unhealthy lifestyles, although potentially preventable, are likely nonetheless. They will incur social and financial costs. It seems almost as certain that the incidence of mental illness will increase over time, leaving doubt as to whether provision will be adequate. Owing to the 'fuzzy' nature of mental illness, however, it is difficult to specify the burden in terms of increasing incidence and cost, especially since poor mental health and physical health are often experienced together. Less certain still is the future of infectious diseases, but planning for them now will limit their impact should they occur. In the context of globalisation this seems increasingly important as a burden of health, and raises a complex set of issues relating to disease control and governance. Finally, there is the related, also uncertain, issue of bio-terrorism. While its risk is probably low, the psychological impact of the perceived threat is more significant and citizens will expect the government to protect them.

Policy recommendations

- The average person living in the UK in the 21st Century potentially faces years of disability, ironically enabled by scientific advance and increased life expectancy. With this comes the associated increase in demand for healthcare and other costs associated with age and morbidity. There is also increasing scope for medical intervention, improved detection and the increased incidence of co-morbidity.
- The broader range of variables that impact on health need to be taken into account, not only focus on lifestyle changes.
- The needs of those with chronic disease imply a blurring of boundaries between the types of care required by individuals – health and social, formal and informal. There is scope to shift the focus from secondary care to primary care, from prevention to cure, to health rather than healthcare.
- It is necessary to establish the overall number of deaths attributable to chronic disease, the spend on chronic disease treatment, and the costs of each chronic disease.
- Mental health service provision would benefit from the development of better detection and early intervention, particularly with high-risk groups, as well as staff training that focuses on the relation between mental and physical health.

- The lack of transparency concerning the resource allocation and actual spending in mental health needs to be addressed.
- Influenza pandemics are inevitable. The most important measure for combating infection is the improvement of integrated surveillance and monitoring systems.
- There is a need to review communicable disease control and public health legislation to ensure that responsibilities are clear and processes are sufficiently robust to be effective in an outbreak or bio-terrorist attack.
- The fear of bio-terrorism represents a greater threat to health than the prospects of the threat itself. A better understanding of the nature of the bio-terrorism threat, an early response plan, a means of dealing with mass casualties and, when possible, an adequate stock of vaccines, a system to manage risk perception even if the threat seems unlikely, and an adequate disease control system are all essential to manage this threat.
- Future UK health policy needs to be located more explicitly in a global context, with opportunities for sharing information and know-how. This is most obvious in the case of disease control, but also in the context of strategies to combat chronic disease such as obesity.

References

AD2000 Collaborative Group (2004) Long-term donepezil treatment in 565 patients with Alzheimer's disease (AD2000): randomised double-blind trial. *The Lancet.* **363**(9427): 2105–15.

Amos B (2004) Mental Health. http://www.publications.parliament.uk/pa/ld199900/ldhansrd/pdvn/lds04/text/40714–04.htm#40714–04_head0. Accessed: 20 July 2004.

Arksey H (2003) Scoping the field: services for carers of people with mental health problems. *Health and Social Care in the Community.* **11**(4): 335–44.

Ashton D (2004) Food advertising and childhood obesity. *Journal of the Royal Society of Medicine.* **98**(2): 51–2.

Ashworth M, Godfrey E, Harvey K and Darbishire L (2003) Perceptions of psychological content in the GP consultation – the role of practice, personal and prescribing attributes. *Family Practice.* **20**(4): 373–5.

Asthma UK (2004) Severe asthma symptoms and ways to control them. Fact Sheet 37. http://www.asthma.org.uk/about/factsheet37.php. Accessed: 22 July 2004.

Audit Commission (1994) *Finding a Place: a review of mental health services for adults.* Audit Commission, London.

Balicer RD, Huerta M and Grotto I (2004) Tackling the next influenza pandemic. *British Medical Journal.* **328**: 1391–2.

Barclay WS (2004) Pandemic risks from bird flu. *British Medical Journal.* **328**: 238–9.

Batty D (2004) Reid unveils chronic care plans. *The Guardian.* 11.3.04.

BBC (2004a) Britons 'ignoring' dementia signs. http://news.bbc.co.uk/1/hi/health/3852557.stm. Accessed: 20 July 2004.

BBC (2004b) Depression pills 'too accessible'. http://news.bbc.co.uk/1/hi/health/3579635.stm. Accessed: 20 July 2004.

BBC (2004c) UK lags on Alzheimer's care. http://news.bbc.co.uk/1/hi/health/3774147.stm. Accessed: 20 July 2004.

BBC News (2004) GPs get new anti-depressant rules. http://news.bbc.co.uk/1/hi/health/4071145.stm. Accessed: 15 December 2004.

Beaglehole R and McMichael AJ (1999) The future of public health in a changing global context. *Development.* **42**(4): 12–16.

Beaglehole R and Yach D (2003) Globalisation and the prevention and control of non-communicable disease: the neglected chronic diseases of adults. *The Lancet.* **362**: 903–8.

Beauchamp DE (2001) Public health as social justice. In: W Teays and L Purdy (eds) *Bioethics, Justice & Health Care.* Thomson Learning, London, pp. 20–3.

Bhopal R (2004) *Questions regarding the disease chapter.* Personal Communication. Email to: Chang, L.

Bloomfield S (2005) Britain worst in EU for heart disease, with costs of £7.5bn a year. *Independent on Sunday,* London. 13.2.05.

BMA (2003) *Adolescent Health.* British Medical Association, Board of Science and Education, London.

BMJ (2004) Minerva. *British Medical Journal.* **328**: 1574.

Bosanquet N and Sikora K (2004) The economics of cancer care in the UK. *The Lancet Oncology.* **5**(9): 568–74.

Boseley S (2003) 50,000 children taking antidepressants. *The Guardian,* London. 20.9.03.

Boyle P, d'Onofrio A, Maisonneuve P, Severi G, Robertson C, Tubiana M and Veronesi U (2003) Measuring progress against cancer in Europe: has the 15% decline targeted for 2000 come about? *Annals of Oncology.* **14**: 1312–25.

British Heart Foundation (2004a) True cost of heart disease. http://www.bhf.org.uk/professionals/index.asp?secondlevel=70&thirdlevel=344&artID=3227. Accessed: 21 May 2004.

British Heart Foundation (2004b) *Coronary Heart Disease Statistics: factsheet.* British Heart Foundation Research Group, Oxford.

Brocklehurst R and Costello J (2003) Health inequalities: the Black Report and beyond. In: J Costello and M Haggart (eds) *Public Health and Society.* Palgrave Macmillan, Basingstoke, pp. 42–60.

Brundtland GH (2004) *Ex-WHO chief sees pay-off in public health worldwide.* Personal Communication. Email to: Portland's World Affairs Council.

Buckley F and Cohen E (2002) Bush to order smallpox vaccinations for military. http://edition.cnn.com/2002/HEALTH/12/11/bush.smallpox/. Accessed: 2 April 2004.

Bunker J (2001) *Medicine Matters After All: measuring the benefits of medical care, a healthy lifestyle, and a just social environment.* The Nuffield Trust, London.

CBI and DH (1992) *Promoting Mental Health at Work.* Confederation of British Industry and Department of Health, London.

Collin J and Lee K (2003) *Globalisation and Transborder Health Risk in the UK: case studies in tobacco control and population mobility.* London School of Hygiene and Tropical Medicine, London.

Communicable Disease Surveillance & Response (CSR), Centre on Global Change and Health and The Nuffield Trust (2004) *Estimating the Impact of the Next Influenza Pandemic: enhancing preparedness.* World Health Organization, Geneva.

Connely J and Emmel N (2003) Preventing disease or helping the struggle for emancipation: does professional public health have a future? *Policy and Politics.* **31**(4): 556–76.

Cooper C and Cartwright S (1996) *Mental Health and Stress in the Workplace: a guide for employers.* The Health and Safety Executive, London.

Cowper A (2004) A New Data Dawns. *Health Service Journal.* **114**: 12–13.

Craig TKJ and Boardman AP (1997) ABC of mental health: common mental health problems in primary care. *British Medical Journal.* **314**: 1609.

Crimmins EM (2001) Mortality and health in human life spans. *Experimental Gerontology.* **36**: 885–97.

de Grey ADNJ (2001) UK research on the biology of ageing. *Experimental Gerontology.* **37**: 1–7.

DfES (2004) *What Works in Promoting Children's Mental Health: the evidence and the implications for Sure Start local programmes.* Department for Education and Skills, Nottingham.

DH (1998) *Modernising Mental Health Services: safe, sound and supportive.* Department of Health, London.

DH (2000) *The NHS Cancer plan: a plan for investment, a plan for reform.* Department of Health, London.

DH (2001) *A National Service Framework for Older People.* Department of Health, London.

DH (2004a) A better life for people with chronic disease. http://www.dh.gov/publicationsand statistics/pressreleasesnotices/fs/en?CONTENT-ID=4076123&chk=5Qt6MX. Accessed: 16 March 2005.

DH (2004b) *Choosing Health: making healthier choices easier. Cmnd 6374.* Department of Health, London.

DH (2004c) *Draft Mental Health Bill. Cmnd 6305–1.* Department of Health, London.

DH (2005) *Supporting People with Long Term Conditions: an NHS and social care model to support local innovation and integration.* Department of Health, London.

DHPE (2004) Addressing infectious disease threats. http://www.astdhpphe.org/infect/infectintro. html. Accessed: 4 October 2004.

Doblhammer G and Kytir J (2001) Compression or expansion of morbidity? Trends in healthy-life expectancy in the elderly Austrian population between 1978 and 1998. *Social Science & Medicine.* **52**: 385–91.

Donelly PD (2004) *Investment in Prevention and the Contribution of Population Health Policy to Improving Health Outcomes.* United Kingdom – Australia Seminar. Federalism, Financing and Public Health. Old Parliament House, Canberra, Australia, Australia Government, Department of Health and Ageing, The Health Foundation, The Nuffield Trust, Australia and London.

Dooley D (2003) Unemployment, underemployment, and mental health: conceptualizing employment status as a continuum. *American Journal of Community Psychology.* **32**(1–2): 9–20.

Dyer L (2004) US judge halts compulsory anthrax vaccination for soldiers. *British Medical Journal.* **329**: 1062.

Ebrahim S and Smith GD (1997) Systematic review of randomised controlled trials of multiple risk factor interventions for preventing coronary heart disease. *British Medical Journal.* **314**: 1666.

European Commission (2003) European Centre for Disease Prevention and Control. http:// europa.eu.int/comm/health/ph_overview/strategy/ecdc/ecdc_en.htm. Accessed: 30 March 2004.

European Commission (2004) Mental Health. http://europa.eu.int/comm/health/ph_determinants/ life_style/mental_health_en.htm. Accessed: 30 March 2004.

Ferrie JE, Shipleya MJ, Stansfeldb SA, Smith GD and Marmota M (2003) Future uncertainty and socioeconomic inequalities in health: the Whitehall II study. *Social Science & Medicine.* **57**(4): 637–46.

Fleck F (2004) Drug industry is not tackling threats to public health, says WHO. *British Medical Journal.* **329**: 1256.

Fontaine KR, Redden DT, Wang C, Westfall AO and Allison DB (2003) Years of life lost due to obesity. *Journal of American Medical Association.* **289**: 187–93.

Foot C (2004) *Questions regarding the burden of cancer.* Personal Communication. Email to: Chang, L.

Frieden TR (2003) Can tuberculosis be controlled? *International Journal of Epidemiology.* **32**: 894–9.

Fries JF (1980) Aging, natural death, and the compression of morbidity. *New England Journal of Medicine.* **303**: 130–6.

Furedi F (2002) *Culture of Fear: risk-taking and the morality of low expectation.* Continuum, London.

Gostin LO (2001) Health promotion and the first amendment: government control of the informational environment. *Millbank Quarterly.* **79**(4): 547–78.

Gray DP (2004a) *Comments on draft burden of disease*. Personal Communication. Email to: Chang, L.

Gray DP (2004b) *Reference*. Personal Communication. Email to: Chang, L.

Greenberg B (1998) *Study shows risk of rare disorder from flu vaccine is slight*. http://www.cnn.com/HEALTH/9812/18/flu.vaccine.ap/index.html. Accessed: 2 April 2004.

Halliwell E (2004) A new mental health taskforce – will health primary care deliver on its potential. *Health Service Journal*. **114**: 25.

Halpern D, Bates C, Beales G and Heathfield A (2004) *Personal Responsibility and Changing Behaviour: the state of knowledge and its implications for public policy*. Prime Minister's Strategy Unit, London.

Halpern D and Cockayne A (2004) *Trust, Engagement and Legitimacy in Public Institutions: summary of interim analytical report*. Cabinet Office, London.

Health Education Authority (1998) *The UK Smoking Epidemic: deaths in 1995*. Health Education Authority, London.

Health Evidence Network (2004a) What are the arguments for community-based mental health care? http://www.euro.who.int/HEN/Syntheses/mentalhealth/20030903_3. Accessed: 27 February 2005.

Health Evidence Network (2004b) What is the evidence on effectiveness of capacity building of primary health care professionals in the detection, management and outcome of depression? http://www.euro.who.int/HEN/Syntheses/capdepr/20041208_2. Accessed: 5 March 2005.

Health Evidence Network (2005) Are disease management programmes (DMPs) effective in improving quality of care for people with chronic conditions? http://www.euro.who.int/eprise/main/WHO/Progs/HEN/Syntheses/DMP/20030820_1. Accessed: 3 February 2005.

Herrman H (2001) The need for mental health promotion. *Australian and New Zealand Journal of Psychiatry*. **35**(6): 709–15.

Hill TP (1996) Health care: a social contract in transition. *Social Science & Medicine*. **43**(5): 783–9.

Hillsdon M, Foster C, Naidoo B and Crombie H (2004) *The Effectiveness of Public Health Interventions for Increasing Physical Activity Among Adults*. Health Development Agency, London.

Holland WW (2002) A dubious future for public health. *Journal of the Royal Society of Medicine*. **95**: 182–8.

House of Commons Health Committee (2004) *Obesity. Third report of session 2003–04*. House of Commons Health Committee, London.

ILC (2002) *Living Longer: healthy to the end?* Longevity and the compression of morbidity. International Longevity Centre Conference 2002, International Longevity Centre, London.

Imperial Cancer Research Fund Oxcheck Study Group (1995) Effectiveness of health checks conducted by nurses in primary care: final results of the Oxcheck study. Imperial Cancer Research Fund. *British Medical Journal*. **310**: 1099–104.

IOM (2003) *Informing the Future: critical issues in health*. Institute of Medicine, Washington DC.

Joint Committee on the Draft Mental Health Bill (2004) Call for evidence. http://www.parliament.uk/parliamentary_committees/jcdmhb.cfm. Accessed: 4 January 2005.

Joint Committee on the Draft Mental Health Bill (2005) *Joint Committee on the Draft Mental Health Bill – First Report*. The United Kingdom Parliament, London.

Jureidini JN, Doecke CJ, Mansfield PR, Haby MM, Menkes DB and Tonkin AL (2004) Efficacy and safety of antidepressants for children and adolescents. *British Medical Journal*. **328**: 879–83.

Kawachi I, Kennedy B and Lochner K (1997) A Long Live Community: social capital as public health. *The American Prospect*. **35**: 56–9.

Kazarian SS, McCabe SB and Joseph LW (1997) Assessment of Service Needs of Adult Psychiatric Inpatients: a systematic approach. *Psychiatric Quarterly*. **68**(1): 5–23.

Kelly CNM and Stanner SA (2003) Diet and cardiovascular disease in the UK: are the messages getting across? *Proceedings of the Nutrition Society*. **62**(3): 583–9.

Kelly MP (2004) *The Evidence of Effectiveness of Public Health Interventions – and the implications*. NHS, Health Department Agency, London.

King's Fund (2001) *General Election 2001 Briefing. Rationing Health Care*. King's Fund, London.

Lalonde M (1974) *A New Perspective on the Health of Canadians*. Ministry of National Health & Welfare, Ottowa.

Langham S, Thorogood M, Normand C, Muir J, Jones L and Fowler G (1996) Costs and cost-effectiveness of health checks conducted by nurses in primary care: the Oxcheck study. *British Medical Journal*. **312**: 1265–8.

Last JM (2001) *A Dictionary of Epidemiology*. Oxford University Press, Oxford.

Lazzari S and Stohr K (2004) Avian influenza and influenza pandemics. *Bulletin of the World Health Organization*. **82**(4): 242–3.

Lehtinen V (2003) Establishment for indicators for mental health monitoring in Europe 1999–2001. http://europa.eu.int/comm/health/ph_determinants/life_style/mental/docs/ev_20031125_co04_en.pdf. Accessed: 30 March 2005.

Leowski J (1998) Essential Public Health Functions: their place in the health-for-all policy for the 21st century. *World Health Statistics Quarterly*. **51**(1): 55.

Lewis R and Dixon J (2004) Rethinking management of chronic diseases. *British Medical Journal*. **328**: 220–2.

Locker D (2003) Living with Chronic Illness. In: G Scambler (ed.) *Sociology as Applied to Medicine*. Saunders, Edinburgh, pp. 79–91.

Lopez AD and Murray CCJL (1998) The global burden of disease 1990–2020. *Nature America*. **4**(11): 1241–3.

Louria DB (2000) Emerging and Re-emerging Infections: the societal determinants. *Futures*. **32**: 582–3.

MacLehose L, Coker R and McKee M (2004) Chapter 13: Communicable disease control: detecting and managing communicable disease outbreaks across borders. In: M McKee, L MacLehose and E Nolte (eds) *Health Policy and European Union Enlargement*. Open University Press, Maidenhead, pp. 185–97.

Marmot M (2004) *Status Syndrome: how your social standing directly affects your health and life expectancy*. Bloomsbury, London.

Martens P (2002) Health transitions in a globalising world: towards more disease or sustained health. *Futures*. **34**(7): 635–78.

McCallum J (1999) The new morbidity picture: substitution versus compression? In: W Bruen and F Proctor (eds) *Compression of Morbidity*. Department of Health and Aged Care, Canberra, Australia.

McCallum J (2001) Health in the 'grey' millennium: romanticism versus complexity? *International Journal of Law and Psychiatry*. **24**: 135–48.

McDaid D (2003) Mental health economics European network: a brief overview. http://europa.eu.int/comm/health/ph_determinants/life_style/mental/docs/ev_20031125_co02_en.pdf. Accessed: 30 March 2004.

McEwan B (2004) *Interview about Stress and Poverty*. BBC, London.

McLean S and Mason JK (2003) Mental health and mental capacity. In: S McLean and JK Mason (eds) *Legal & Ethical Aspects of Healthcare*. GMM, London, pp. 211–24.

Mental Health Foundation (2004a) Mental health problems. http://www.mentalhealth.org.uk/page.cfm?pagecode=PMMH. Accessed: 17 May 2004.

Mental Health Foundation (2004b) *Time for Public Mental Health: a briefing from the Mental Health Foundation in advance of the White Paper on public health*. Mental Health Foundation, London.

Monaghan S (2004) Illuminate the debate. *Health Service Journal*. **114**: 18–19.

Monaghan S, Huws D and Navarro M (2003) *The Case for a New UK Health of the People Act*. The Nuffield Trust, London.

Montgomery J (2003) Public health law. In: *Public Health*. Oxford University Press. Oxford, pp. 23–50.

Morgan M (2003) Hospitals and patient care. In: G Scambler (ed.) *Sociology as Applied to Medicine*. Saunders, Edinburgh, pp. 66–77.

Morgan OWC, Griffiths C and Majeed A (2004) Association between mortality from suicide in England and antidepressant prescribing: an ecological study. *BioMed Central Public Health*. 4(1): 63.

Murphy E (2004) Case management and community matrons for long-term conditions. *British Medical Journal*. **329**: 1251–2.

NHS (2003) *The NHS Cancer Plan: three year progress report – maintaining the momentum*. Department of Health, London.

NHS Hertfordshire (2004). Mental Health. http://www.nhsinherts.nhs.uk/hp/health_topics/mental_health/mental_health.htm. Accessed: 20 July 2004.

Nickell LA, Crighton EJ, Tracy CS, Al-Enazy H, Bolaji Y, Hanjrah S, Hussain A, Makhlouf S and Upshur REG (2004) Psychosocial effects of SARS on hospital staff: survey of a large tertiary care institution. *Canadian Medical Association Journal*. **170**: 793–8.

Nicoll A and Hamers FF (2002) Are trends in HIV, gonorrhoea, and syphilis worsening in western Europe? *British Medical Journal*. **324**: 1324–7.

ONS (2003a) *Mental Health of Older People*. National Statistics, London.

ONS (2003b) HIV and AIDS: 53 000 people living with HIV in the UK. http://www. statistics.gov.uk/cci/nugget.asp?id=654.

Opinion Leader Research (2004) *Public Attitudes to Health Policy*. King's Fund, London.

Pajak S, Mears A, Kendall T, Katona C and Medina J (2003) *Workload and Working Patterns in Consultant Psychiatrists: an investigation into occupational pressures and burdens report*. Royal College of Psychiatrists, London.

Palmer SR, Salmon RL, Thomas DR, Morgan M, Smith MM and Bartlett CLR (1999) *The Contribution of Global Health Policy to the Control of Emerging Infectious Diseases. Implications for the UK*. The Nuffield Trust, London.

Parkes J (2004) *Questions re CDM*. Personal Communication. Email to: Chang, L.

Parliamentary Office of Science and Technology (2001) *Postnote: bio-terrorism*. Parlimentary Office of Science and Technology, London.

Pink D and Prior C (2004) Power to the people. *Health Service Journal*. **114**:16–17.

Poole R, Ryan T and Pearsall A (2002) The NHS, the private sector, and the virtual system. *British Medical Journal*. **325**: 349–50.

PPA (2003) PPA: News – pact pages. http://www.ppa.org.uk/news/pact-112003/pact-112003.htm. Accessed: 7 October 2004.

Price D, Pollock AM and Shaoul J (1999) How the WTO is shaping domestic policies in health care review. *The Lancet*. **354**(9193): 1889–92.

Rankin J (2004) *Developments and Trends in Mental Health Policy*. Institute for Public Policy Research, London.

Raphael D (2003) Barriers to addressing the societal determinants of health: public health units and poverty in Ontario, Canada. *Health Promotion International*. 18(4): 397–405.

Riemsma RP, Pattenden J, Bridle C, Sowden AJ, Mather L, Watt IS and Walker A (2003) Systematic review of the effectiveness of stage based interventions to promote smoking cessation. *British Medical Journal*. **326**: 1175–7.

Rothman AA and Wagner EH (2003) Chronic illness management: what is the role of primary care? *Annals of Internal Medicine*. **138**(3): 256–61.

Sausman C (2003) The future health workforce: an overview of trends. In: C Davies (ed.) *The Future Health Workforce*. Palgrave Macmillan, London, pp. 222–41.

Sikora K, Bosanquet N and Slevin M (2005) *Cancer Care in the NHS*. Reform, London.

Singh D (2004) New infectious diseases will continue to emerge. *British Medical Journal*. **328**: 186.

Singh-Manoux A, Adler NE and Marmot MG (2003) Subjective social status: its determinants and its association with measures of ill-health in the Whitehall II study. *Social Science & Medicine*. **56**(6): 1321–33.

Smith A (2001a) European infectious disease surveillance – think big! *British Medical Journal*. http://bmj.bmjjournals.com/cgi/eletters/323/7317/818#16960.

Smith A (2001b) A healthy colour. *The Guardian*. 25.4.01.

Sweeney KG, Macauley D and Gray DP (1998) Personal significance: the third dimension. *The Lancet*. **351**: 134–6.

Tanne JH (2004) Depression affects elderly people's lives more than social illness. *British Medical Journal*. **329**: 1307.

The Economist (2001) Avoiding a dark winter. http://www.economist.com/displaystory.cfm?story_id=835123. Accessed: 4 April 2005.

The Economist (2003) Who will build our biodefences? http://www.economist.com/displaystory.cfm?story_id=1560369. Accessed: 4 April 2005.

The Economist (2004) Drug problem. http://www.economist.com/displaystory.cfm?story_id=2620194. Accessed: 27 May 2004.

The Royal College of Psychiatrists (2005) The living project. http://www.rcpsych.ac.uk/cru/hsrp/Livingwithseriousmentalilllness.htm. Accessed: 4 April 2005.

The Sainsbury Centre for Mental Health (2003) *Briefing 22. Money for Mental Health: a review of public spending on mental health care*. The Sainsbury Centre for Mental Health, London.

The Wellcome Trust (2004) *Public Health Sciences: challenges and opportunities. Report of the Public Health Sciences Working Group convened by the Wellcome Trust*. The Wellcome Trust, London.

Thomas CM (2003) Cost of depression among adults in England in 2000. *The British Journal of Psychiatry*. **183**: 514–19.

Timimi S (2004) Rethinking childhood depression. *British Medical Journal*. **329**: 1394–8.

Trueland J (2004) 'Instead of looking at my disability, listen to what I'm trying to tell you'. *Health Service Journal*. **114**: 21.

Turner HT (2004) Long-term outcome of treating schizophrenia. *British Medical Journal*. **329**: 1059.

Unwin C, Blatchley N, Coker W, Ferry S, Hotopf M, Hull L, Ismail K, Palmer I, David A and Wessely S (1999) Health of UK servicemen who served in the Persian Gulf War. *The Lancet*. **353**(9148): 169–78.

Vallgarda S (2001) Governing people's lives. *European Journal of Public Health*. **11**(4): 386–92.

Wagner EH (2000) The role of patient care teams in chronic disease management. *British Medical Journal*. **320**: 259–72.

Wanless D (2002) *Securing our Future Health: taking a long-term view*. HM Treasury, London.

Wanless D (2003) *Securing Good Health for the Whole Population: population health trends*. HM Treasury, London.

Wanless D (2004) *Securing Good Health for the Whole Population. Final Report*. HM Treasury, London.

White M (2004) Yesterday's man provides much-needed wisdom on NSF. *Health Service Journal*. **114**: 21.

WHO (2001a) *Mental Health: new understanding, new hope*. World Health Organization, Geneva.

WHO (2001b) Statement to the press by the Director-General of the World Health Organization, Dr Gro Harlem Brundtland: World Health Organization announces update guidance on smallpox vaccination. http://www.who.int/inf-pr-2001/en/state2001-16.html. Accessed: 2 April 2004.

WHO (2003a) *Mental Health in the WHO European Region: Fact sheet EURO/03/03*. World Health Organization, Copenhagen.

WHO (2003b) Fact sheet no. 211: Influenza. http://www.who.int/mediacentre/factsheets/fs211/en/. Accessed: 15 December 2004.

WHO (2004a) Fact sheet no. 104: Tuberculosis. http://www.who.int/mediacentre/factsheets/fs104/en/. Accessed: 4 October 2004.

WHO (2004b) Fact sheet: Avian influenza. http://www.who.int/mediacentre/factsheets/avian_influenza/en/. Accessed: 6 April 2004.

WHO Medicines and Policy Department (EDM) (2004) *Priority Medicines for Europe and the World Project: 'a public health approach to innovation'*. World Health Organization, Geneva.

Wilkinson D, Stave C, Keohane D and Vincenzino O (2004) The role of general practitioners in the diagnosis and treatment of Alzheimer's disease: a multinational survey. *Journal of International Medical Research*. **32**(2): 149–59.

Wilkinson RG (1996) *Unhealthy Societies: the afflictions of inequality*. Routledge, London.

Wilson D and Bhopal R (1998) Impact of infection on mortality and hospitalisation: a study in the North East of England. *Journal of Public Health*. **20**: 386–95.

Wood B (1999) The politics of health. In: B Jones (ed.) *Political Issues in Britain Today*. Manchester University Press, Manchester and New York, pp. 150–64.

Woodward S and Ramsey R (2004) Body matters. *Health Service Journal*. **114**: 35.

Yach D (2004) *Lecture in Chronic Disease*. The Nuffield Trust, London.

Yach D and Hawkes C (2004) *WHO Long-term Strategy for Prevention and Control of Leading Chronic Diseases*. World Health Organization, Geneva.

Yuen P (2000) *OHE Compendium of Health Statistics*. Office of Health Economics, London.

Chapter 7

Where will technology take us?

Zoë Slote Morris and Don E Detmer

This chapter discusses possible changes in technology relevant to UK health in 2020 and how policy can both influence and be influenced by them. Rather than attempting to forecast developments, it identifies areas of potential change and considers implications for public policy. Focusing on healthcare technology and its adoption, it provides snapshots of technological developments, highlighting areas for possible policy change. The first section looks at medical technology, including drugs, genetics, tissue engineering, miniaturisation and process technology, and the second section examines information technology, including telemedicine and 'e-health'.

Medical technology

Medical technology can be defined as:

> *The drugs, devices and medical and surgical procedures used in medical care and the organisation and supportive systems within which such care is provided (US Office of Technological Assessment, 1982).*

This definition makes explicit the difference between product technology and process technologies, which describe the way in which (or where) technical tasks are performed.

Future developments

'In the area of scientific and technology discoveries ... future projections are often over optimistic about what will be discovered by when and make unrealistic assumptions about the implementation of discoveries in everyday use' (Bloom *et al.*, 2000). Attempts have been made to forecast the future (Foresight, 2000; Marinker and Peckham, 1998; Peckham, 2000b; Sykes, 2000; Wild and Torgesen, 2000; Wilson, 1999), but there is inevitably a trade-off between 'earlier warning and greater accuracy' (Robert *et al.*, 1998). Some over-prediction results from unexpected occurrences (Peckham, 2000b), some from focusing on what is technically possible rather than what is ethically desirable or socially possible (Kendall, 2001).

Technological discovery, innovation and application are social processes, contingent on social and political choices. Understanding possible technological changes – and the processes that promote or inhibit their development – is essential for policy formulation and advocacy regarding the trajectory of a technology or innovation. The take-up and application of technologies (adoption and diffusion) vary, not just with the health needs of a given community and technological possibility, but according to 'political, economic, religious, cultural, social or legal factors' (Mays, 1993). The UK has tended to embrace product technologies more slowly than comparator nations, arguably because of the way in which healthcare is funded and the associated cost containment (Mays, 1993). While slower adoption is not always a bad thing – and some current technologies prove unbeneficial, even damaging, in the longer term (Glied, 2003) – there is a tension in policy between attempting to grow the UK health technology industry (HM Treasury *et al.*, 2004), and attempting to contain costs and thereby being 'less receptive' as a purchaser (DTI, 2003). New technology is typically associated with higher costs (Fuchs, 1996; Glied, 2003; Newhouse, 1992), although these can be offset by health improvements (Cutler and McClellan, 2001).

Current health policy places increasing importance on identifying and assessing new technologies (Dargie, 2000) through the National Health Service Research and Development Programme, the Health Technology Assessment (HTA) programme, guidance based on evaluations from the National Institute for Clinical Excellence (NICE), increased focus on evidence-based medicine (EBM) and the implementation of National Service Frameworks (NSFs). NSFs are not evaluated by NICE (Maynard *et al.*, 2004). These aim to improve healthcare provision and outcomes and to support a more standardised service.[1]

It is crucial that policymakers and managers attempting to introduce new technologies understand what determines adoption and diffusion. Williamson (1992) suggests that the sort of knowledge leading to the take-up of new technologies can be 'knowledge-driven' or 'problem-solving'. NICE guidance and NSFs assume an optimal solution to a problem which may differ from current provision (Berg, 2002) and that take-up is knowledge-driven. There is considerable evidence, however, that 'robust, scientific evidence, of itself is insufficient to ensure diffusion' (Fitzgerald *et al.*, 2002). Individuals are more likely to apply new knowledge if they believe in it and think that they need it. Thus, clinicians may discount evidence they consider irrelevant to their particular patients or care settings (Fitzgerald *et al.*, 2002). Professional subgroups have different notions of 'credible' sources and different definitions of what 'knowledge' is. Clinicians, for instance, tend to rely overly on randomised control trials (HITF, 2004).

Although the process of adoption tends to be conceived of as linear, in practice it involves innovation and iteration (Mays, 1993). New technologies are not adopted in a vacuum – they are considered against factors such as financial incentives and patient demands. Fitzgerald *et al.* (2002) suggest that 'in healthcare … networks are one of the key determinants of whether an innovation is successfully diffused or not'. Effective networks are characterised by trust and respect. A need to cross professional and organisational boundaries where, for instance, there is unequal status between groups may inhibit adoption.

---

[1] Implementation of NICE guidelines, for example, is found to vary by trust and clinical area (Sheldon *et al.*, 2004). New measures will require the Healthcare Commission to rate trusts on implementing NICE guidelines (HSJ, 2004c). This does not address the wider discussions around the application of guidelines (for example, Dent and Sadler, 2002; Summerton, 2004). NICE guidelines are not always consistent with 'best evidence', or existing guidelines based on such evidence, or accurate – for example managing hypertension (Poulter, 2004), or evidence-based medicine more generally (*see* for example, Guyatt *et al.*, 2004 on EBM and patient values).

Denis and Langley (2002) suggest that 'the way in which ... benefits and risks maps on to the interests, values, and power distribution of the adopting system (organisation, inter-organisational group, sets of professionals) is critical to understanding the way in which innovations diffuse'. 'A practice community may be reluctant to accept the efficacy of a novel treatment because it threatens their status or professional position' (Fitzgerald *et al.*, 2002). There is, therefore, an argument for user involvement in the development of guidance, if new practices are to be implemented.[2] Thus, the 'capacity of an organisation to innovate will depend upon the history, culture and quality of relationships and these will vary by context' (Fitzgerald *et al.*, 2002). Additional factors can include the ease of adoption and local enthusiasm, as well as external factors such as media campaigns, manufacturers' inducements and government regulations (Stevens *et al.*, 1997).[3]

Drugs

Infections continue to pose a threat to human health, especially when associated with increased resistance. There have not been any new classes of anti-microbial drugs introduced in the last 20 years, nor are any anticipated until 2007 (Peckham, 2000a). The Standing Medical Advisory Committee (SMAC) found that 75% of antibiotics were of 'questionable value' (SMAC, 1997). Moreover, there is an increase in drug-resistant bacteria.

The massive global pharmaceutical industry is 'ailing' as the introduction of new 'blockbuster' drugs slows (*The Economist*, 2004a). 'About 50 new drugs are launched each year' (Stevens *et al.*, 1999) but particular drugs are effective in only about 30% of patients. This could force pharmaceutical firms to place more emphasis on developing drugs with smaller markets. McKinnon *et al.* (2004) dispute the claim that 'Big Pharma' is struggling, either in terms of compounds or earning potential overall for the future. They anticipate decline in the launch of 'blockbusters'. Pharmacogenetics, discussed further below, is another field certain to influence market dynamics in the future.

Orphan drugs, used to treat rare diseases, are less profitable and therefore not a natural area of development for pharmaceutical companies. To address this market failure, the EU Regulation on Orphan Medical Products (141/2000) was passed in 1999. It defined a rare disease as one that affected less than five per 10 000 of the population, and provided incentives designed to encourage the development of drugs for rare diseases. Products will be allowed a ten-year period of market exclusivity, and a possible reduction or waiver in registration fees. Member states may provide additional incentives, such as R&D support and tax breaks. Similar legislation in the US is associated with increased development.[4] The National Horizon Scanning Centre reports an increase in the number of orphan drugs

---

[2] 'Rigidly determined, scientifically-based guidelines will not always mesh with good clinical judgement; and there may be conflict between the goal of managing costs and both guidelines and clinical judgement' (Callahan, 1999). Guidelines need to be sensitive to social differences.

[3] The introduction of lithotripsy was slow in France because the government waited for French-made machines to become available. They were also very slow to adopt 'in-and-out', 'day' or 'ambulatory' surgical operations.

[4] Between 1983 and 1994, 600 orphan products were developed, compared with ten in the decade before the Orphan Drug Act.

reaching the EU market (Packer, 2004).[5] Policy that creates incentives and allows barriers to persist can have a major impact on technological innovation.

The cost of providing appropriate incentives remains uncertain. In the above example incentive costs include implementation, lost tax revenue and the high prices predicted for drugs associated with small markets. EU regulations, through the Committee for Orphan Medicinal Products (COMP), will address 'excessively profitable' products. Although evidence from the US suggests these products are rare (four excessively profitable products defined so far), there will be complexities in defining excess profit and how to deal with it. As pharmacogenetic research clarifies smaller and smaller disease categories and populations, companies may limit the indications for particular drugs to afford them 'orphan status'. There may also be issues in evaluating a product with a small sample size. A fine balance is needed between providing incentives necessary for orphan drug development and ensuring that the industry is supported and sensibly regulated (Karr, 2000). This is a common tension in technological development.

From an economic perspective, both in terms of industrial development and cost savings in healthcare, it is worth making the effort to develop regulation which is appropriate (HITF, 2004). Some issues, however, lie beyond the control of the UK government. There are concerns, for example, that the Clinical Trials Directive (designed to protect volunteers in trials) will have a 'catastrophic' effect on small trials, rendering university research dependent on large pharmaceutical companies (Tomlinson, 2004).

Genetics

Genetics is the study of single genes and their effects. Genomics refers to the study of the functions and interactions of all genes in the genome, including their contribution to health (Guttmacher and Collins, 2003). Pharmacogenetics applies genomic knowledge to drug discovery. Also relevant to the practical application of genetics in health are proteomics, transcriptomics, glycomics and metabolomics (*The Economist*, 2003).[6] In such a complex arena, making specific futures forecasts is difficult. Developments in one area of technology are contingent on others, for example, developments in genetics will also depend on the availability of IT.

It is anticipated that advances in genetics will support four areas of healthcare: prevention and diagnosis, including screening; therapy; enhancement; and reproduction. Early diagnosis is expected to improve the management of a disease and, in the case of carriers, inform reproduction choices. There are already tests that predict predispositions to breast cancer, haemochromatosis, colon cancer and melanoma (Peckham, 2000a).

---

[5] *See* European Commission (2005) for EU drugs registered for human use since 2000.
[6] A gene is a set of DNA letters that has all the information required to make a protein. It includes instructions about the beginning and end of the protein (punctuation) and where and when to make the protein. Proteomics refers to 'cataloguing and analysing ... the protein molecules produced in an organism'. Transcriptomics describes 'logging the intermediary molecules, known as RNAs, that carry information from the DNA in the nucleus to the rest of the cell'. Glycomics involves logging carbohydrate molecules that may influence how the proteins work. Metabolmics is used to describe the process of studying the 'small molecules that are processed by proteins' (*The Economist*, 2003).

Most current diagnoses relate to rare but devastating monogenetic disorders. Since gene therapy will be expensive (one US estimate is $100 000 per patient), this raises ethical questions regarding efficacy, cost-effectiveness and equity (Mendelsohn, 1999). Most therapies cost less over time, and so initial costs should not be seen as reflecting costs once a technology is more widely available.

Genetic screening of populations could identify people 'at risk' of particular diseases and allow appropriate interventions to be introduced before the disease develops (Ginsburg and McCarthy, 2001). This should shift the role of medicine away from 'crisis-driven intervention to predictive medicine' (Khoury *et al.*, 2003) and from treating the symptoms of disease to eliminating its cause (Ginsburg and McCarthy, 2001; Reiss, 2001). This approach towards preventative medicine or 'prospective' medicine (Snyderman and Williams, 2003) is embodied in the White Paper *Our Inheritance, Our Future: realising the potential of genetics in the NHS* (DH, 2003b).

Health services will most likely need to refocus on 'maintaining wellness, moving away from the present operation of a "sickness service"; from palliatives to prevention' (Sykes, 2000). The 'individualisation of medicine' will 'feed in to [patients'] push for control over their own care', thereby supporting more tailored health-promotion intervention (Sykes, 2000). It is not clear why public health messages would be any more effective for people with a genetically-determined, as opposed to behaviourally-determined, risk; nor how this will fit in with policy issues of equity and personal responsibility. Population screening is less acceptable to today's public than is seeking a monogenetic disorder diagnosis (Durant, 1999).

'Therapeutic and preventative benefits arising from the discovery of genes could lag 20 to 50 years behind the diagnosis' (Cantor, 1992). This raises questions regarding the appropriateness of diagnosis and screening if no novel treatments are available (Nelkin, 1992).[7] The prediction based on genes is still imperfect and the notion of 'risk' is not a simple one (Innovative Health Technologies, 2003). In these 'early days' genetic testing imposes a burden of worry and powerlessness on some 'patients' and makes additional demands on the healthcare workforce to educate and counsel.[8] This has resource implications, as does increased monitoring (Peckham, 2000b).

To date, little testing for monogenetic disorders is carried out in the private sector, not least because the Advisory Committee on Genetic Testing (ACGT) voluntary code of practice requires firms to provide counselling. This increases costs and makes the service less attractive to commercial providers. Instead tests are carried out in Regional Genetics Centres – in 1998–99 approximately 43 000 genetic tests were undertaken in NHS genetics laboratories (Expert Working Group to the NHS Executive and Human Genetics Commission, 2000).

---

[7] This has broader implications. For example, Krantz *et al.* (2004) argue that screening for herpes virus type 2, for which there is currently no treatment, is unethical on several grounds, including beneficence and justice.

[8] One proposal from the *Our Inheritance, Our Future* White paper (DH, 2003b) is a new Genetics Education and Development Centre to spearhead education and training in genetics for all healthcare staff, with more genetic services expected to be carried out in primary care. Robins and Metcalfe's (2004) study of Australian GPs suggests that 'cognitive deficit', that is lack of information about genetics, is less of an issue than GP's desire to locate genetics care in the more holistic context. They want access to information on a need-to-know basis, which they can relate to specific patients. They do not want general education on genetics.

There is evidence of huge potential public demand for such services. Frost and Sullivan (2001, cited in Martin and Frost, 2003) estimate a US market worth $200 million by 2006 for predisposition testing. The recent provision of tests by Sciona through The Body Shop and the Internet signals a receptive UK public, albeit for 'lifestyle' tests (BBC, 2002).

Ultimately, gene therapy will mean the replacement or deletion of a defective somatic (adult) gene to eliminate the associated illness. Since this has been little developed, it is unlikely to have a profound effect on UK health in 2020. Relph *et al.* (2004) note that while there have been successes, in the treatment of Severe Combined Immunodeficiency (SCID), for example, the number of people having treatment is small and the process of using viral vector still potentially problematic. Kimmelman (2005) provides a useful review of some of the technical risks and ethical concerns associated with gene transfer and considers some policy implications.

More challenging from an ethical perspective is the use of gene therapy to eliminate future disease by means of germ line manipulation – that is by changing the genes in cells that are transmitted from one generation to the next. Currently the technology is not available, but some people question whether the development is actually necessary when other interventions are available (Mendelsohn, 1999) or if it will ever be considered ethical.

The US Institute of Medicine of the National Academies states that while somatic gene therapy is ethically no different to other therapy, germ line enhancement and eugenic engineering is unique, 'since tampering with germ lines touches the very essence of human development' (Nicholas, 1988, quoted in Mendelsohn, 1999). Attitudinal research suggests that the general public has clear views on what is and what is not acceptable, and there appears to be a belief that this will shape how the field develops (Abbott, 1998, cited by Kent, 1999; Stratford *et al.*, 2001a,b).

The use of gene therapy for 'enhancement' is currently considered to be unacceptable but the definitions of a medical condition versus 'enhancement' are not clear-cut. Homosexuality was once considered to be a medical condition, and could again be potentially amenable to 'treatment' if there is a 'gay' gene (Hamer and Copeland, 1999).[9] In Europe, it appears that what is considered acceptable relates more to existing moral attitudes than to assessments of risk. Risk, moral acceptability and potential benefits are offset against each other as the public assesses overall acceptability (Durant, 1999). Baylis and Robert (2004) present 11 reasons for genetic enhancement being ethically unsound but contend that it is inevitable nonetheless.

The challenge for policymakers is to forge agreement between different standpoints, while ensuring effective legislation and regulation that reflect community views. Some argue that public perceptions of science are too conservative (meaning too risk-averse).[10] In developing views, consideration needs to be given to the 'fuzzy' nature of acceptable boundaries and the uncertain relationship that 'novelty' has always had in scientific developments when seen through the eye

---

[9] Data from the British Social Attitudes Survey revealed that 18% of respondents said that changing a person's genes should 'definitely' or 'probably' be allowed to 'make a person straight, rather than gay or lesbian' (and 6% gay rather than straight) (Stratford *et al.*, 2001a).

[10] Research on stakeholder perceptions of each other as well as GM food, for example, revealed high levels of mismatch (Marris *et al.*, 2002).

of the public.[11] Stratford *et al.* (1999) also find that public attitudes towards genetics are embedded within attitudes to science more generally – whether it 'does more harm than good'. This points to the problem of identifying 'a public' for engagement and education.

Pharmacogenetics

A less problematic extension of genetics is pharmacogenetics, that is using genetic testing to guide prescribing based on an understanding of interactions between an individual's genetic constitution and drugs, or the genetic nature of their disease (Weinshilboum, 2003). Lymphomas which look identical can be genetically different (Lemonick, 2000) and this information could explain why only some people respond to 'appropriate' treatment (Detmer and Steen, in press). The current TRANSBIG trial in Brussels, for example, aims to identify 'microarray data' predicting which breast cancer patients need chemotherapy after surgery. This could relieve some women of 'unnecessary and unpleasant' treatment (*The Economist,* 2004b).

Commercial firms are actively pursuing pharmacogenetics because it is expected to improve their product development. Currently, 'of all compounds entering preclinical development, about 90% fail prior to launch' (Sykes, 2000), often due to lack of knowledge about how particular compounds behave in the body. Better understanding of genetic determinants of disease and metabolisation of drugs will allow pharmaceutical companies to conduct more efficient development and trials. It will also enable companies to market drugs to people who will not suffer the side-effects associated with particular compounds. Pharmacogenetics should support more accurate and efficient prescribing. Genelex, for example, already sells tests direct to customers over the Internet to assess how well individuals metabolise a range of commonly-used drugs (Genelex, 2005).

A recent study of pharmacogenetics concluded that the 'introduction of pharmacogenetic "products" is likely to be gradual, but a majority [of experts] believed that pharmacogenetics could have an impact on the care of more than 15% of patients within 15 years [2018]' (Melzer *et al.*, 2003). There are concerns, however, that drug companies may focus on diseases with the most common molecular structures, or that the resulting compounds may be more expensive owing to their smaller markets (*The Economist,* 2004b). It is also recognised by the industry that 'developing new chemical drugs is proving harder than expected' (DTI, 2003).

Even if development is slow, it will be disruptive to current healthcare arrangements. Genetics has the potential to redefine 'disease', 'treatment' and 'patients', demanding new relationships with 'patients'. Other relevant issues include the psychological consequences for individuals and their families of finding out that they carry or might develop a disease, informed consent, issues around privacy and access, confidentiality and concerns about the use of information by employers and insurers (Lenaghan, 1998; Martin and Frost, 2003; Peckham, 2000b; Stratford *et al.*, 2001a,b). The Genetics and Insurance Committee's (GIAC) 2000 ruling, allowing the use of some genetics tests by insurance companies, makes the UK 'particularly

---

[11] Witness the fascination and ambivalence as exemplified by Frankenstein and related science fiction movies.

permissive' in this regard, and runs counter to public attitudes, and there may be a further question regarding whether the public will be willing to pay for more individualised treatment (*The Economist*, 2004b).

Progress in genetic testing has accelerated. This is especially true of diagnostic testing, much of which occurs in the commercial sector, sometimes too quickly for regulatory bodies to keep up (Martin and Frost, 2003). Recent attempts to have Sciona withdraw its products from the UK high street revealed gaping holes in current regulatory arrangements. The Human Genetics Commission (HGC), although critical of the scientific validity and information provided to customers by Sciona, did not publish its report for fear of legal action by the company (whose products were not covered by existing regulations since they qualify as consumer products).

The issue of regulation in general is not straightforward. There is a tension between providing an environment in which commercial developments can flourish and safeguarding citizens. The HGC recognises a need for consistency across different types of tests, including genetic tests. It also acknowledges a trade-off between the potential psychological damage caused by genetic information, and the right of individuals to such information (HCG, 2002, cited in Martin and Frost, 2003). The nature of genetic information is not strictly 'personal' since it may also reveal information about other people who are currently alive (Hope, 2004). Martin and Frost (2003) suggest a range of regulatory responses including licensing, a role for NICE in assessment and legislation against genetic discrimination. This is a two-way process, as regulatory choices will impact on the development of new technologies:

> if policymakers decide that all predisposition testing is potentially 'dangerous' and should be linked to genetic counselling, then this will give the NHS and the medical profession a monopoly over these tests, limit the role of firms as direct service providers and restrict how much information is available to the public. Alternatively, if most genetic tests are seen as being unexceptional and similar to diagnostics that can be bought over the counter in pharmacies [e.g. cholesterol tests, sperm count tests, pregnancy tests], then the cases for medical control and state intervention are much more limited. Under the latter conditions, a larger market for testing and personal genetic information may emerge (Martin and Frost, 2003).

This is important in terms of predicting future developments because it points to the dilemma facing policymakers. While they have an interest in encouraging commercial genetic research – both biotechnology and pharmaceuticals are significant players in the UK economy (Strategy Unit, 2003), with the DTI estimating the biotechnology industry to have a market capitalisation of £18 billion in 2000 – departments purchasing health technologies will be concerned by spiralling costs. Reconciling these views will be difficult. According to *The Economist*, 'The uncertainty over regulatory and public reaction is one of the reasons why, over the past four years, at least two dozen firms working to create transgenic animals have gone bust. Most of these were in Europe' (*The Economist Technology Quarterly*, 2004).

Estimating cost implications associated with genetics is not clear. Some anticipate savings (Bell, 1997; Sykes, 2000), others do not (Zimmern and Cook, 2000). The net impact is impossible to discern today since some gains are certain to be offset by some losses and early results may bear little resemblance to circumstances when technologies mature. It could be that the impact of screening on public health has cost benefits and developments in pharmacogenetics may allow existing drugs, previously dismissed as too toxic or ineffective, to find use in particular sub-populations.

If a private firm patents a gene and asserts the associated entitlement, it is likely to result in an expensive test. This in turn will drive up health costs or exclude people from treatment (Martin and Frost, 2003). Matthijs (2004) suggests that some US laboratories are not offering diagnostic tests for hemochromatosis because they are too expensive. Cancer Research UK, on the other hand, has patented BRCA2 genes but allows public European laboratories to use them without charge. Since the use of free licences does not reward the innovator, Matthijs (2004) argues rather in favour of having genes exempted from the European Patent Convention. He suggests this would allow more access to diagnostics, while providing commercial protection for developing more costly therapeutics. Issues pertaining to the patenting and licensing of genes are currently being discussed internationally. The majority of the public feels that genetic information should be publicly owned and available, despite the investment of commercial organisations. This would have obvious implications for future technological development (HCG, 2002, cited in Martin and Frost, 2003).

The complexity and cost associated with clinical genetics suggest that practical progress may be slow, and the impact may not become evident until around 2020. Some regard this as fortuitous, since it allows time for policy and ethics to 'catch up' (Mendelsohn, 1999). Others believe that law and policy will forever lag behind unless they encase biotechnology in such a net of 'red tape' that research becomes impossible.[12]

Tissue engineering

Tissue engineering is another area of increasing technological significance. It involves combining human cells with synthetic biomaterials to create products such as skin, cartilage, bones and organs. Tissue engineering rests on the use of stem cells. These are 'master cells', which can develop into any type of other cell, and replicate many times over a long period to grow new tissue. Certain kinds of somatic stem cells appear to specialise in or differentiate between particular conditions and also to group, potentially allowing tissues and organs to be developed from our own cells. They provide a perfect match with our bodies, reducing the risk of rejection. Potentially, it could help alleviate the shortage of donor organs for transplantation.[13]

---

[12] In a speech to the Royal Society in 2002, Tony Blair drew attention to this point by saying 'When I was in Bangalore in January, I met a group of academics who were also in the business of the biotech field. They said to me bluntly: "Europe has gone soft on science; we are going to leapfrog you and you will miss out"' (quoted in Wilsdon and Willis, 2004).

[13] The number of transplanted organs increased by 3% in 2003–04, but lists are still long (HSJ, 2004b). Whilst some biotech companies are attempting to develop genetically modified animals for xenoplantation, there are serious ethical concerns with the public, as well as worries about the transmission of disease across species (zoonotic infections) (*The Economist Technology Quarterly,* 2004). The real concern is that, once moved from animals to humans, infections continue to spread to humans. Given these difficulties, it may be that development in new mechanical devices has greater contribution to make to rehabilitation (Poole-Wilson, 1998).

It has been claimed that stem cell development will grow blood (BBC, 2001d), new teeth *(The Economist,* 2004c), fingers (Personal, 1999a), neuroprecursor cells affected by Alzheimer's (BBC, 2001a), kidneys (BBC, 2001b), hearts (BBC, 2001c) and bone marrow, as well as repairing stroke damage. Researchers at the University of Liverpool are currently using it to address Age-related Macular Degeneration (AMD), of which 15 000 new cases are expected next year (Faculty of Medicine, 2005). Scientists in Australia, for example, are 'close' to making a sphincter made from tissue from another part of a patient's body. Developers believe it will make a significant contribution to the wellbeing of incontinent people in ten years' time, given the imperfections of current alternatives.

Thus, tissue engineering, although still in the development phase, has huge potential given the health needs of an ageing population. Optimists argue, 'In 2020, we will have made substantial progress towards true "cloning" of certain organs, but many difficult technical steps will remain before successful cloning of a heart or a lung' (Drell and Adamson, 2003). Since human stem cells were only extracted in 1998 – 20 years after the extraction of stem cells from mice (NIH, 2002) – it is likely to be some time before usable organs are produced. Developments are restricted by knowledge of long-term stability of new tissue and the tendency of somatic stem cells to differentiate towards particular cells (Vats *et al.,* 2004). Besides slow progress in science, ethical issues arise regarding the use of stem cells. A UN decision on calls for a complete global ban on cloning, for example, is continually delayed (Linton, 2005; Mayor, 2004a,b).

Britain is the first western country to license cloning *(The Economist,* 2004d). In England, the current Human Tissue Act (2004) was modified in the final stages 'to allow research using material from living patients without consent but with safe-guards' (Dyer, 2004). The bill did not differentiate between tissue acquired by surgery or post-mortem, nor between different types of tissue (Furness and Sullivan, 2004). Consent is meant to be 'explicit', although actual mechanisms are not specified. Furness and Sullivan estimate that the time taken to inform, get consent and input the relevant data for an average year would translate to 2680 jobs – the equivalent of two medium-sized NHS hospitals. This points to the difficulty of getting regulation right. An additional risk in tight regulation is the outward migration of the scientific workforce.

Miniaturisation (including nanotechnology)

As miniaturisation becomes easier to use and more applicable, the scope for diagnosis and treatment at home (self-care) and in primary care is likely to increase. Rashid (2000) identified a range of miniaturised devices likely to be introduced into primary care in the next 'two to three years' which would reduce the need for referral, as well as the wait for test results. Increasing ease of use could lower screening costs, improve outcomes and lower use of secondary care, resulting in increased patient satisfaction and greater access to services. Questions remain as to whether improved diagnosis would increase the demand for secondary care beyond its ability to cope, and how much this would cost. Supporters argue that, based on the experience with other diseases, screening is beneficial to health service costs because it reduces treatment costs in the longer term (Rashid, 2000). There is evidence that good management of a chronic illness, such as diabetes, can significantly reduce costs by avoiding early development of expensive complications of the disease (Rashid, 2000).

Associated with miniaturisation is the increased application of implantable devices. These devices will have an impact on diagnostics and the early delivery of therapy. The recent HITF report (2004) describes a closed-loop insulin management device incorporating blood sugar sensors and delivery for use with diabetes. Recently featured in the *Health Service Journal* are devices such as a cardiac resynchronisation therapy (CRT) implant used to synchronise the contractions of both heart ventricles. Already available and effective, it is seen as the forerunner of similar systems designed to manage chronic illness. Imperial College, London is developing devices designed to monitor young people at risk of cardiac arrhythmia (UbiMon), and seniors at home (UbiSense). UbiSense involves multiple low-cost wireless infrared-based sensors being used to monitor the health status of an individual through analysing his/her gait, posture and activities (Darzi, 2004). The development of these technologies allows people suffering from chronic disease to remain out of hospital and more active, benefiting patients while reducing costs.

Nanotechnology refers to research and technology at the atomic, molecular or macromolecular level. It has unique functionality due to its size.[14] Although nanotechnologists are probably premature in their claims for its potential (Stix, 2002), which includes the abolition of some diseases (Drexler, 1987), it is in limited use already in products such as water softeners and sun-tan lotion. The US National Science Foundation estimates that the nanotechonology industry could be worth $1 trillion by around 2018 (Ratner and Ratner, 2003). Likely nanotechnological applications in healthcare include: better research science (Boyd, 2003); safer, more efficient drug development; drugs which only treat target cells through physical implantation (Langer, 2003); tissue engineering at the molecular level (Wood *et al.*, 2003); better diagnostic testing (Ratner and Ratner, 2003); and the extension of existing application of neural implants to allow computers to be linked to the human nervous systems (Kurzweil, 1999).

A meeting (2003) of the Royal Society and the Royal Academy of Engineering discussed what nanotechnologies would become available in the near future and what would delay developments. Anticipated hold-ups to 'biotechnology and nanomedicine' relevant to contemporary policy included: lack of interdisciplinary funding for research, lack of new funding, a low skills base amongst staff (partly because of nanotechnology's interdisciplinary nature), a need for 'big science' infrastructure, a need for close links with industry and universities, and public perceptions.[15] Although largely ignorant, the public worry about 'messing with nature', for example (Royal Society and Royal Academy of Engineering, 2003).[16] There is increasing recognition that some 'bridging' of communities needs to occur,

---

[14] Generally between one and 100 nanometers.

[15] Similar barriers to development are identified in The Academy of Medical Sciences' report *Strengthening Clinical Research* (2003). Such barriers include lack of facilities and infrastructure, lack of trained staff, inadequate funding for trials, a failure to use the opportunities for research offered by the NHS and the increasingly complex bureaucratic, legal and ethical systems of the UK and EU.

[16] An Economic and Social Research Council (ERSC) study provides a useful summary of the economic and social implications of nanotechnology (Wood *et al.*, 2003).

as well as more 'upstream' engagement – that is, in the design phase – if nanotechnology is to avoid becoming 'the next GM' (Wilsdon and Willis, 2004).[17] Similarly, early developments will not produce obvious consumer benefits and improved profits are more likely to irritate than inspire consumers (*The Economist*, 2004e). Moreover, some 'grey goo' fears have foundations in reality: there is little knowledge about the toxicological risks of nanotechnology and self-replication. As with the patenting of genes, there are also concerns over who might own nanotechnologies. Besides the specific policy issues mentioned by the Royal Society and the Royal Academy of Engineering, matters common to most of the new forms of technology outlined here – ensuring adequate regulation, patient protection and public education – are relevant to nanotechnology too.

Process technologies

Crucial to many new technologies is the idea of innovation in process. For example, non-invasive techniques are providing useful advances in cardiology to provide better diagnostic information and to guide treatment (Prasad *et al.*, 2004). It is likely that minimal invasive surgery (MIS) practice as it currently stands represents the tip of the iceberg. At present application is uneven (Sedrakyan *et al.*, 2004b), even where there is evidence of improved outcomes (Sedrakyan *et al.*, 2004a). This indicates the need to consider social aspects in the implementation of new processes (McCulloch, 2004). Genetic and non-genetic screening will result in patients seeking advice and possible treatment in the pre-disease stage. They may find MIS more acceptable (and possible) than gene therapy (Darzi, 2004).

Developments in process are contingent on developments in other areas of technology. Thus, IT is associated with greater potential use of telesurgery, robotics (including telerobotics) and Master Slave Manipulators and micro-electro-mechanical systems (MEMS). The development of anaesthetic substitutes is also likely to impact significantly on process.

ICT, telemedicine and e-health[18]

> *The health sector's most avoidable shortcomings can be linked to data ... Lost data, poor documentation, lack of access to available knowledge, and reliance on memory all impede the delivery of high quality healthcare services. Public health agencies lack the ability to share critical information quickly and encounter substantial difficulties when attempting to pool existing data for analysis. Advances in medical knowledge and treatment capabilities often take too many years to reach patients; many therapeutic interventions in use are not supported by evidence of effectiveness. Practice patterns differ across institutions and regions, resulting in varying health outcomes and costs of care. Patients trying to make*

---

[17] Nanotechnology is one area being funded under the DTI's £2.1 million grant scheme to help scientists, industry and policymakers to engage with the public (DTI, 2004).

[18] Telemedicine refers to the use of IT to shorten physical distance. E-health is variously defined as any health-oriented activity that uses IT, or health activities specifically engaging consumers or patients themselves, typically linking the patient with professional care-givers.

informed health decisions often encounter conflicting information with varying degrees of quality. And, care delivery is often extraordinarily wasteful of patients' time (Detmer, 2003).

The US Institute of Medicine identifies six direct uses for IT in healthcare:

- consumer health (including lay education)
- clinical care
- administration and finance
- public health
- research
- professional education.

These are not mutually exclusive categories since information infrastructures with the correct architecture can assure that patient health records can feed into public health records and support professional education and research, for example. Telemedicine crosses several of these functional boundaries and is discussed below.

E-health or consumer health

E-health or consumer health refers to citizens' and patients' use of IT, largely enabled by the spread of Internet access. There is evidence that patients increasingly use the Internet to check doctors' advice covertly, to develop expertise and to gather information about diseases that are embarrassing to talk about (Ziebland *et al.*, 2004).

  This has policy implications in terms of the changing roles of clinicians, patients and informal carers and regarding the quality of information on the Internet. Some argue that the explosion of information available to patients is potentially disabling. It could place new demands on GPs as 'brokers' required to translate general information for individual relevance (Berg, 2002). With an increasing emphasis on self-care and a more 'engaged' patient, heavy reliance on the Internet is likely to bring about greater divisions in society in the short term since there are clear demographic differences in Internet use (Golding, 2000). Some argue that such inequalities are not inevitable, but need managing (Ziebland *et al.*, 2004). Indeed, Gustafson *et al.* (2001) have shown with randomised trials that lower educational and socio-economic levels do not equate with poorer IT capabilities if managed appropriately.

  In 2012, the UK will switch to Digital Interactive Television. The potential this offers goes far beyond simply using the TV as an Internet device. Direct personalised advice and contact with health practitioners will be possible through the TV, with potential to transform health.

Clinical care

The NHS Information Authority plans to introduce electronic patient records (EPRs) by 2005. The electronic patient record[19] is akin to current medical records

---

[19] An associated idea is personal health records, which will allow individuals to monitor and track information relevant to maintaining their own health.

that hold information on indications and treatment,[20] although in addition the electronic form will hold records of allergies, treatment histories and test results. It should be useable across the range of health settings, including social care and by high street pharmacists.[21] When combined with robust evidence-based adaptive decision-support protocols embedded within the electronic health record (EHR), substantial gains could be made, if not impeded by incompatibility of GP and hospital IT systems (*The Times*, 2005). According to the Department of Health, 90% of GPs regularly use computers for clinical care. Fernando *et al.* (2004) suggest, however, that 'the safety features of ... systems currently in use in about three-quarters of UK practices have clinically important deficiencies', and better supplier information is needed.

Between 4 and 12% of hospital admissions are estimated to result from adverse drug advents.[22] EPRs should reduce this figure. Bates *et al.* (1998) already show the dramatic benefits of such technology for improving the safety and efficacy of drug delivery in hospital settings. IT can improve healthcare delivery through: alerts (high and low lab. values); assistance in drug choices and dosages; calculations and suggestions (adjusting mechanical ventilators, for example); critiques (rejecting an order); diagnosis and reminders (Geissbuhler and Miller, 2000) and computer-generated prescriptions (Alemi *et al.*, 1996).[23]

Berg (2002) argues that if patients 'own' their records then they are entitled to access, remove and modify things that are written about them.[24] Although health-care workers need complete data, knowing that patients have access to records will encourage them to modify their recording and perhaps spawn a parallel 'informal' system. The general challenge for policymakers is balancing demands for more information with the need for privacy and confidentiality.

Administration and finance

In the US, information and communications technology has contributed most clearly in the past to administrative and financial transactions (Turban *et al.*, 1996, cited in Committee on Quality of Health Care in American, IOM, 2001). Although the latter is currently of less significance in the UK, saving on administration will be

---

[20] From the perspective of the GP, NICE protocols could be implemented on wireless handheld devices by GPs which would transform the diagnosis and referral processes. More procedures could be undertaken by para-professional staff, for example nurse practitioners and pharmacists and the scope for improved self-diagnosis and home care could be greatly extended.

[21] The US Food and Drug Administration has recently approved an implantable device which, when scanned, reveals a patient's unique identifier number, allowing teams to access records 'on a secure database via encrypted internet access' (Tanne, 2004).

[22] According to the *BMJ*, 'the cost to the NHS of adverse drug reactions leading to hospitalisation [is] £470 million a year' (Eaton, 2004).

[23] Computer-generated prescriptions (11% errors) are eight times more accurate than hand-written prescriptions according to a recent hospital-based study (Young *et al.*, 2004; Committee on Quality of Health Care in America, IOM, 2001). Paper prescriptions will be phased out in England from 2005. An evaluation report suggests some implementation issues related to software, business processes and 'negative attitudes' (Watts, 2004).

[24] Nearly all legal systems mandate that the formal medical record can be amended but not modified. That means that substitute language cannot be replaced by erasing the original information. Rather, records can be amended to offer corrections or additions or different points of view.

substantial given the estimate that a quarter of time is spent managing information (Wyatt, 1995, cited in Peckham, 2000b), with disease management and legal require-ments certain to increase. It should also reduce the problem of mislaid notes and missing results, recognised by policymakers ten years ago (Audit Commission, 1995a,b).

As policy in England moves towards 'payment by results' (PBR) better recording of activity will be essential. The same is true of delivering improved quality in the NHS. Currently 'inconsistent and highly contested data throw the whole of the Quality Agenda into a confusing fray' (Leatherman and Sutherland, 2003). An electronic staff record is currently being piloted on three sites, although a timetable for roll-out has not been announced (HSJ, 2004a). Furthermore, as the delivery of care is taken on by a broader range of providers, patients and carers will need information regarding who provides which services.

Public health and research

If person-specific information is removed, patient records have the potential to be aggregated and so generate sets of community data, allowing population studies to be carried out. Consent, confidentiality and technical issues may arise, however, and an information system designed to support delivery of healthcare may not be of direct use for research purposes and vice versa (Garrod, 1998, cited in Berg, 2002). Creating datasets that are useful for delivery and research functions requires additional work, increasing the cost of inputting data.

Integration of patient data prompts difficult questions in terms of who sees the data and who is responsible for it. Ironically, more oversight lessens information privacy. This is especially complex when the whole point of integration is to support the flow of data across boundaries. As Wyatt and Keen (2001) have argued, 'sharing data requires clinicians to trust one another, and non-clinical colleagues, far more than is common at the moment'. The *Information Strategy for IT* does not address the need of sharing data with social care organisations and other organisations outside the NHS (Wyatt and Keen, 2001), despite requiring integrated arrangements for people leaving healthcare for social care under the Care Standards Act (2000). It also does not suggest how to balance these needs with issues of data protection.

There is great value in using clinical data in research, as the new 'clinical roadmap' of the National Institute of Health illustrates (NIH, 2005). For example, 'extraordinary gains' in paediatric cancer care in the US have been attributed 'in part' to treatment centres' participation in clinical trials in which natural data was gathered, analysed and fed back into treatment patterns (Committee on Quality of Health Care in America, IOM, 2001, citing Simone and Lyons, 2000). There is also clear evidence that most people want healthcare teams to have access to data that contribute to their care (Watts, 2004).

The issue of clinical trials does require urgent attention, however, if the unique opportunity to utilise the NHS for research is to be addressed (DTI, 2003). The Department of Trade and Industry's Bioscience Innovation and Growth Team has made a strong case both in terms of economics – one of main drivers of spiralling trials costs being associated with the difficulty in recruiting patients – and in terms of benefits to patient care. Barriers relate to infrastructure and funding, but also to 'a lack of cultural support for innovation ... and collaboration'. Ways of shifting this culture are being explored by policymakers (RPBWP, 2004).

Professional education

The European Working Directive is driving change to the way in which health-workers are trained by opening up workforce markets and increasing the focus on competence-based practice. The physical location of care is also relevant, the greater use of treatment centres and specialists centres for example. These trends in service provision tend to suggest that all levels of medical and non-medical training will be delivered differently, specifically through training technologies such as virtual reality and e-universities (Darzi, 2004).

Despite the potential benefits of better use of IT, it often takes years of investment before there is even a hope of savings being realised (Berg, 2002). Moreover, despite huge injections of cash into this area of the NHS, results have not been encouraging. Reviewing progress in 2002 against the NHS IT strategy (1998), Detmer (2002) concluded that, even after four years, little progress could be seen. The main barrier is people. Bowns *et al.* (1999) suggest that recruiting good IT staff to the NHS is made more difficult since national pay scales cannot compete with commercial salaries. Most people within the NHS are too narrow in their thinking to use IT to redesign their work for safety, efficiency and patient-centred care. Recent estimates of the final cost of implementing the IT programme place them three to five times more than originally declared (from £6.2 million to between £18.6 and £31 billion) (BBC News, 2004).

Bowns *et al.* (1999) note that the NHS is characterised by a series of sub-cultures and an inverted power structure within which managers 'influence' rather than 'control' staff. Staff have shown themselves to be resistant to changes in process, especially if these are believed to threaten status (*see*, for example Jones, 2003). In addition, 'an apparent litany of failed or discredited projects, often centrally led, has left a widespread perception that modern [ICT] and healthcare do not mix' (Bowns *et al.*, 1999). Excessive guidance and commercial disputes have not helped in the past and look set to be repeated (Timmins, 2004).

It is necessary to have appropriate incentives to encourage diffusion (van der Lei *et al.*, 1993). 'Government intervention has been the catalyst for introducing computerisation [in primary care], and financial incentives (e.g. money to purchase equipment and free use) have also been significant' (Pemberton *et al.*, 2003). Yet, this has not occurred within the timescale set by government, evenly across practices or against all the objectives set (*see* Tai *et al.*, 2000). IT is still under-utilised (Gillies, 1998) but this is likely to change gradually in the future, for example with the introduction of electronic booking systems (DH, 2004).

Bowns *et al.* (1999) identify a broader range of issues which need to be recognised and addressed in any IT strategy. These include:

- a need to align corporate, human resources and IT strategies
- a need for changes in process
- commitment from senior managers, competent middle managers and good project management
- a good understanding of change management
- adequate staff training.

On an operational level there needs to be user-involvement, time, money and flexibility to deliver the system (Lorenzi, 2004).

Actual development of IT in healthcare requires 'conscious and careful management of human resources', adequate resources, appropriate measures for security
and confidentiality and agreed standards to allow data to be classified and moved.
Institutions need to commit to transferring and storing data, and place a greater
emphasis on IT (Berg, 2002). The shifting locations of care present additional
challenges in this regard (Keen and Wyatt, 2005; Rigby, 2005).

Telemedicine and telecare

It is anticipated that the use of telemedicine – medicine at a distance, be it education,
monitoring or treatment – will spread in the future.[25] Telemedicine can increase
scope for self-care, and more treatment in primary care. The University of California
Medical Centre is already testing a robot which allows clinicians to check on and
interact with patients from home (Dobson, 2004). Although, as Mays (1993) notes,
telemedicine technology has been available in the UK for 30 years, application has
been modest. This may be due to the UK's small size and dense population (Mays,
1993; Peckham, 2000b).[26] Theoretically, IT should help equalise access to healthcare as proximity to physical services becomes less significant. In Wales, there are
already telegenetics services designed to prevent people travelling long distances to
a 'centre' (Gray *et al.*, 2000).

The most obvious UK examples of telemedicine to date are NHS Direct and NHS
Online. Evaluations of early teleconsultations seem positive (Mair and Whitten,
2000), but with reservations: patients are happy to use telephone and email for
minor problems, but are less confident about more complex and nuanced exchanges
(May *et al.*, 2001). The emergence of the 'expert patient' (Coulter, 2002; Detmer
et al., 2003; DH, 2003a) may alter this dynamic in the future. Concerns that email
'may offer choice but probably at the expense of access' has yet to be addressed
(Wong, 2004). Car and Sheikh (2004) provide a review of the use of email and
guidance on how consultations should be managed,[27] while Ferguson and Frydman
(2004) suggest that making greater use of electronic media in health will require
'something akin to a major system upgrade in our thinking'.

Telemedicine can save patient and clinician time in the secondary setting, and
improve GPs' knowledge. Peckham (2000b) describes a project undertaken at the
Derriford Hospital in Plymouth in 1998. The public accessed 'Molewatch clinics'
through a GP. The image of the moles was transmitted by ISDN link to cancer
specialists who responded in 24 hours. A 100% agreement rate was found between
the assessment of digital images and assessment of the actual mole a week later. The
use of telemedicine was estimated to expedite treatment by one month. It also
improved GPs' knowledge of lesions (Personal, 1999b).

The potential impact of telemedicine on patient satisfaction is likely to be
significant if it supports self-care and primary care: most people would rather go
to their GP than be a hospital outpatient (Bowling *et al.*, 1997) and would prefer to
spend more recovery time at home (Lenaghan, 1998). To realise this potential

---

[25] A useful review of the scope for telemedicine in provided by Norris (2001).

[26] But it need not take place within national boundaries.

[27] 'The ethical considerations, professional etiquette, and legal rules that guide traditional
communication between healthcare professionals and patients are equally applicable to email
consultations' (Car and Sheikh, 2004).

several issues need to be addressed. Besides the need for a robust and usable IT system and the associated issues, effective telemedicine still requires expert staff to provide care.

Telemedicine requires expertise from outside medicine, challenging boundaries and demanding new forms of working. Another issue is payment, as the costs (for example, call centres for monitoring) and savings (for example, emergency calls and wasted visits) fall to different budgets (Brownsell *et al.*, 1999). Where users are seniors, will this be health or social care? Furthermore, while there is evidence that patient engagement in treatment decisions can improve outcomes (Coulter and Rozansky, 2004), such changes are likely to place greater demands on the patient.

Conclusions

The past 20 years have seen huge changes in technological applications in health and the potential for change in the next 20 years is even greater. It is contingent on a range of factors, many of which lie outside science and technology. The NHS is typically a late adopter and slow diffuser, but also has a lot of out-of-date equipment. A recent study by the Liberal Democrats estimated a replacement backlog of £3.14 billion (Burstow, 2004). This point is acknowledged by Wanless (2002) who adds that 'recent central capital initiatives have begun to address this issue ... but mechanisms to upgrade equipment in the future are still not in place'.

If policy is being driven by expectations of cost savings, this will end in disappointment. Historically, medical technology has contributed to an increase in expenditure (Newhouse, 1992), although specific technologies can reduce overall costs, for example through shorter recovery times or reduced levels of hospitalisation (such as The Medical Technology Group 2004). As technology is refined it can be applied to more vulnerable and frequently older groups, and thus also contribute to higher costs by increasing the pool of potential patients (Dozet *et al.*, 2002). Already there are concerns of insufficient money to meet NICE guidance (Burke, 2002). There is evidence to suggest that payment methods influence diffusion (Mays, 1993). There is currently concern from medical technology firms that payment by results in England will limit their domestic markets, damage their businesses and ensure that the UK remains a 'late' adopter. It is questionable whether hospitals operating below the tariff introduced as part of PBR will use the difference to invest in technology.

For policymakers, it is more important to understand the processes by which technology may be hindered or supported than to predict specific technological advances. Below are some general considerations that should aid policy formulation and implementation in the future.

Policy recommendations

- Technology is considered to be vital to the economic health of the UK but there are issues around public–private partnerships.
- Technology development is largely driven by commercial sector investment so is not always appropriate to needs of healthcare and carers. The government could provide incentives for the development of needed technologies.

- There is some urgency to resolve ethical issues – for example, those related to technological developments in genetics and the use of human tissue – with policy responses and legislation. Sound policy should be developed within a clear ethical and legal framework in anticipation of such developments.
- Current and anticipated gaps in regulation should be addressed.
- The notion of 'privacy' needs attention and a structured well-designed public education strategy is overdue.
- Technology is a social phenomenon which has implications for how technology policy is developed.
  - Where the introduction of technology is top-down, appropriate incentives will be essential (for example, with IT in primary care).
  - New technologies will alter the boundaries of care – for example by increasing the scope for self-care. While this can be viewed as a positive change, it will present considerable challenges in its implementation. Within the NHS the problems associated with a need to cross boundaries or change practices must be addressed.
  - New technology will alter the relationship between professionals and patients. It will support decentralisation of care and empowerment through information. Technology could empower or diminish the significance of the patient as agent, although the patient will be better informed with more options for care.
- Progress will be slower, more expensive, and less cost-effective than anticipated; cost savings to the care system may not occur at all but higher levels of safety and quality may improve productivity at the societal level.
- Future developments in medical technology, and their potential impact on health outcomes, are likely to be 'patchy'. There is no clear 'correct' policy path. Choices will be made between 'conflicting goods': privacy versus information; innovation versus regulation; public funding versus private profit; and economic development versus healthcare cost-containment.

References

Academy of Medical Sciences (2003) *Strengthening Clinical Research*. The Academy of Medical Sciences, London.

Alemi F, Allemango SA, Goldhagen J, Ash L, Finkelstein B, Lavin A, Butts J and Ghadiri A (1996) Computer reminders improve on-time immunization rates. *Medical Care*. **34**(10): 45–51.

Audit Commission (1995a) *For Your Information: a study of information management and systems in the acute hospitals*. Audit Commission, London.

Audit Commission (1995b) *Setting the Records Straight*. Audit Commission, London.

Bates D, Leape L, Cullen D, Laird N, Petersen L and Teich J (1998) Effect of computerized physician order entry and a team intervention on prevention of serious medication errors. *Journal of the American Medical Association*. **280**(15): 1311–16.

Baylis F and Robert JS (2004) The inevitability of genetics enhancement technologies. *Bioethics*. **18**(1): 1–26.

BBC (2001a) Breakthrough for stem cell research. http://news.bbc.co.uk/1/hi/sci/tech/1683424.stm. Accessed: 4 April 2004.

BBC (2001b) New hope for kidney patients. http://news.bbc.co.uk/1/hi/health/1454060.stm. Accessed: 4 April 2004.

BBC (2001c) Scientists grow heart cells. http://news.bbc.co.uk/1/hi/health/1468260.stm. Accessed: 4 April 2004.

BBC (2001d) Stem cells turned to blood. http://news.bbc.co.uk/1/hi/sci/tech/1524066.stm. Accessed: 5 March 2004.

BBC (2002) Row over gene testing kit. http://news.bbc.co.uk/1/hi/sci/tech/1868767.stm. Accessed: 26 August 2004.

BBC News (2004) Warning of major NHS IT overspend. http://newsvote.bbc.co.uk/mpapps/pagetools/print.news.bbc.co.uk/1/hi/health/3734504.stm. Accessed: 12 October 2004.

Bell W (1997) *Foundations of Futures Studies*. Transaction Publisher, New Brunswick, NJ.

Berg M (2002) Patients and professionals in the information society: what might keep us awake in 2013. *International Journal of Medical Informatics*. **66**: 31–7.

Bloom BS, Pouvourville N, Libert S and Fendrick AM (2000) Surgeon predictions on growth of minimal invasive therapy: the difficulty of estimating technological diffusion. *Health Policy*. **54**: 201–7.

Bowling A, Stramer K, Dickinson E, Windsor J and Bond M (1997) Evaluation of specialists' outreach clinics in general practice in England: process and acceptability to patients, specialists, and general practitioners. *Journal of Epidemiology and Community Health*. **51**: 52–61.

Bowns IR, Rotherham G and Paisley S (1999) Factors associated with success in the implementation of information management and technology in the NHS. *Health Informatics Journal*. **5**: 136–45.

Boyd RS (2003) Devices watch time (almost) stand still. *Charlotte Observer*. 11.3.03.

Brownsell SJ, Williams G, Bradley DA, Bragg R, Catlin P and Carlier J (1999) Future systems for remote health care. *Journal of Telemedicine and Telecare*. **5**: 141–52.

Burke K (2002) No cash to implement NICE, health authorities tell MPs. *British Medical Journal*. **324**: 258.

Burstow P (2004) http://www.paulburstow.libdems.org.uk.

Callahan D (1999) Remembering the goals of medicine. *Journal of Evaluation in Clinical Practice*. **5**(2): 103–6.

Cantor C (1992) The challenges to technology and informatics. In: D Kevles and L Hood (eds) *The Code of Codes: scientific and social issues in Human Genome Project*. Harvard University Press, Cambridge, MA.

Car J and Sheikh A (2004) Email consultations in health care: 1 – scope and effectiveness. *British Medical Journal*. **329**: 435–8.

Committee on Quality of Health Care in America, IOM (2001) Using information technology. In: R Briere (ed.) *Crossing the Quality Chasm: a new health system for the 21st century*. National Academy Press, Washington DC, pp. 175–92.

Coulter A (2002) *The Autonomous Patient: ending paternalism in medical care*. The Nuffield Trust, London.

Coulter A and Rozansky D (2004) Full engagement in health. *British Medical Journal*. **329**: 1197–8.

Cutler DM and McClellan M (2001) Is technological change in medicine worth it? *Health Affairs*. **20**(5): 11–29.

Dargie C (2000) *Policy Futures for UK Health. 2000 Report*. The Nuffield Trust, London.

Darzi A (2004) *UK Policy Futures: technology*. Personal communication. Email to: Morris, ZS.

Denis J and Langley A (2002) Introduction to forum. *Health Care Management Review*. **27**(3): 32–4.

Dent THS and Sadler M (2002) From guidance to practice: Why NICE is not enough. *British Medical Journal*. **324**: 842–5.

Detmer DE (2002) Building the data and informatics capabilities: the role of information and communications technology in improving quality. (Unpublished paper.)

Detmer DE (2003) Building the national health information infrastructure for personal health, health care services, public health, and research. *BMS Medical Informatics and Decision Making.* **3**(1).

Detmer DE, Singleton PD, MacLeod A, Wait S, Taylor M and Ridgwell J (2003) *The Informed Patient: study report.* Cambridge University Health, Cambridge.

Detmer DE and Steen EB (2005) New technologies and health statistics. In: D Friedman, E Hunter and R Parrish (eds) *Health Statistics: shaping policy and practice to improve the population's health.* Oxford University Press, Oxford.

DH (2003a) *The Expert Patient: a new approach to chronic disease management for the 21st century.* Department of Health, London.

DH (2003b) *Our Inheritance, Our Future: realising the potential of genetics in the NHS.* Cmnd 5791-II. Department of Health, London.

DH (2004) Work under way to set up booking systems. http://www.dh.gov.uk/PolicyAnd Guidance/PatientChoice/WaitingBookingChoice/WaitingBookingChoiceArticle/fs/en?CONTENT _ID=4083786&chk=%2BWT2kT. Accessed: 12 October 2004.

Dobson R (2004) Meet Rudy, the world's first 'robodoc'. *British Medical Journal.* **329**: 474.

Dozet A, Lyttkens CH and Nystedt P (2002) Healthcare for the elderly: two cases of technology diffusion. *Social Science & Medicine.* **54**(1): 49–64.

Drell D and Adamson A (2003) Fast forward to 2020: what to expect in molecular medicine. Accessed: 2 March 2004.

Drexler KE (1987) *Engines of Creation: the coming era of nanotechnology.* Anchor Books, New York.

DTI (2003) *Bioscience 2015. Improving National Health, Increasing National Wealth.* Department of Trade and Industry, Bioscience Innovation and Growth Team, London.

DTI (2004) New grant scheme launched to encourage greater public engagement with science. http://www.gnn.gov.uk/Content/Detail.asp?ReleaseID=128594&NewsAreaID=2. Accessed: 8 September 2004.

Durant J (1999) Public understanding of the significance of genomics. In: P Williams and S Clow (eds) *OHE Conference on Genomics, Healthcare and Public Policy.* Office of Health Economics, London, pp. 23–32.

Dyer C (2004) Human Tissue Bill is modified because of research needs. *British Medical Journal.* **328**: 1518.

Eaton L (2004) More surveillance of drugs is needed to protect public. *British Medical Journal.* **329**: 1124.

European Commission (2005) Community register of medicinal products for human use. http:// pharmacos.eudra.org/F2/register/alfregister.htm#h255. Accessed: 31 March 2005.

Expert Working Group to the NHS Executive and Human Genetics Commission (2000) *Laboratory Service for Genetics.* Department of Health, London.

Faculty of Medicine (2005) Experimental ophthalmology unit. http://www.liv.ac.uk/clinical sciences/root/experimental%20ophthalmology%20unit/index.htm. Accessed: 4 April 2005.

Ferguson T and Frydman G (2004) The first generation of e-patients. These new medical colleagues could provide sustainable healthcare solutions. *British Medical Journal.* **328**: 1148–9.

Fernando B, Savelyich BSP, Avery AJ, Sheikh A, Bainbridge M, Horsfield P and Teasdale S (2004) Prescribing safety features of general practice computer systems: evaluation using simulated test cases. *British Medical Journal.* **328**: 1171–2.

Fitzgerald L, Ferlie E, Wood M and Hawkins C (2002) Interlocking interactions, the diffusion of innovations in health care. *Human Relations.* **55**(12): 1429–49.

Foresight (2000) *Healthcare.* Foresight, London.

Fuchs V (1996) Economics values and health care reform. *American Economic Review.* **86**(1): 1–24.

Furness P and Sullivan R (2004) The human tissue bill. *British Medical Journal.* **328**: 533–4.

Geissbuhler A and Miller RA (2000) Computer-assisted clinical decision support. In: GB Chapman and FA Sonnenberg (eds) *Decision Making in Health Care: theory, psychology and applications.* Cambridge University Press, Cambridge.

Genelex (2005) DNA testing leaders. http://www.genelex.com. Accessed: 4 April 2005.

Gillies A (1998) Computers and the NHS: an analysis of their contribution to the past, present and future delivery of the National Health Service. *Journal of Information Technology.* 13: 219–29.

Ginsburg GS and McCarthy JJ (2001) Personalized medicine: revolutionized discovery and patient care. *Trends in Biotechnology.* 19: 491–6.

Glied S (2003) Health care costs: on the rise again. *Journal of Economic Perspectives.* 17(2): 125–48.

Golding P (2000) Forthcoming features: information and communications technologies and the sociology of the future. *Sociology.* 34(1): 165–84.

Gray J, Brain K, Iredale R, Alderman J, France E and Hughes H (2000) A pilot study of telegenetics. *Journal of Telemedicine and Telecare.* 6: 245–7.

Gustafson DH, Hawkins R, Pingree S, McTavish F, Arora NK, Mendenhall J, Cella DF, Serlin RC, Apantaku FM, Stewart J and Salner A (2001) Effect of computer support on younger women with breast cancer. *Journal of General Internal Medicine.* 16(7): 435–45.

Guttmacher AE and Collins FS (2003) Ethical, Legal, and Social Implications of Genomic Medicine. *The New England Journal of Medicine.* 349(6): 562–9.

Guyatt G, Cook D, and Haynes B (2004) Evidence based policy making is about taking decisions based on evidence and the needs and values of the population. *British Medical Journal.* 329: 988–9.

Hamer DH and Copeland P (1999) *Living with Our Genes: why they matter more than you think.* Macmillan, London.

Healthcare Industries Task Force (2004) *Reports from working groups and overview of key recommendations (Draft).* HITF, London.

HM Treasury, Department of Trade and Industry and Department of Education and Skills (2004) *Science & innovation investment framework 2004–2014.* HM Treasury, London.

Hope T (2004) *Medical Ethics: A Very Short Introduction.* Oxford University Press, Oxford.

HSJ (2004a) E is for Electronic Staff Record. *Health Service Journal.* 114: 39.

HSJ (2004b) in brief. *Health Service Journal.* 114: 8.

HSJ (2004c) Merger must not hamper implementation. *Health Service Journal.* 114: 3.

Innovative Health Technologies (2003) *Delivering and Experiencing Innovative Health Technologies: Users' Perspectives.* Innovation Health Technologies, 3rd Annual Meeting. University of York, York.

Jones M (2003) 'Computers can land people on Mars, why can't they get to work in hospitals?' Implementation of an Electronic Patient Record System in a UK Hospital. *Methods of Information in Medicine.* 42: 410–15.

Karr A (2000) Who wants to adopt an orphan? *Hospital Pharmacist.* 7(6): 165–7.

Keen J and Wyatt J (2005) The social epidemiology of information technologies. In: S Dawson and C Sausman (eds) *Future Health Organisations and Systems.* Palgrave Macmillan, London.

Kendall L (2001) *The Future Patient.* Institute for Public Policy Research, London.

Kent A (1999) *Patient's perspectives.* OHE Conference on Genomics, Healthcare and Public Policy. Office of Health Economics, London, pp. 51–7.

Khoury MJ, McCabe LL and McCabe ERB (2003) Population screening in the age of genomic medicine. *New England Journal of Medicine.* 348: 50–8.

Kimmelman J (2005) Recent development in gene transfer: risk and ethics. *British Medical Journal.* 330: 79–82.

Krantz I, Lowhagen G-B, Ahlberg BM and Nilstun T (2004) Ethics of screening for asymptomatic herpes virus type 2 infection. *British Medical Journal*. **329**: 618–21.

Kurzweil R (1999) *The Age of Spiritual Medicines*. Viking, New York.

Langer R (2003) Where a pill won't reach. *Scientific American*. **288**: 50–7.

Leatherman S and Sutherland K (2003) *The Quest for Quality in the NHS. A Mid-Term evaluation of the Ten-Year Quality Agenda*. The Nuffield Trust, London.

Lemonick MD (2000) *The genome is mapped. Now what?* http://www.time.com/time/archive/preview/0,10987,997338,00.html. Accessed: January 2002.

Lenaghan J (1998) *Brave New NHS? The impact of the new genetics on the health service*. Institute for Public Policy Reseach, London.

Linton L (2005) *U.N. Group Calls For Cloning Ban*. http://www.cbsnews.com/stories/2004/10/21/tech/main650621.shtml. Accessed: 18 February 2005.

Lorenzi N (2004) Beyond the gadgets: Non-technological barriers to information systems need to be overcome too. *British Medical Journal*. **328**: 1146–7.

Mair F and Whitten P (2000) Systematic review of studies of patient satisfaction with telemedicine. *British Medical Journal*. **320**: 1517–20.

Marinker M and Peckham M (1998) *Clinical Futures*. British Medical Journal Books, London.

Marris C, Wynne B, Simmons P and Weldon S (2002) *Public Perceptions of Agricultural Biotechnologies in Europe. Final Report of the PABE research project summary*. Centre for the Study of Environmental Change, University of Lancaster, Lancaster.

Martin P and Frost R (2003) Regulating the commercial development of genetic testing in the UK: problems, possibilities and policy. *Critical Social Policy*. **23**(2): 186–207.

Matthijs G (2004) Patenting genes may slow down innovation, and delay availability of cheaper genetic tests. *British Medical Journal*. **329**: 1358–60.

May C, Mort M, Mair FS and Williams T (2001) Factors affecting the adoption of telehealthcare technologies in the United Kingdom: the policy context and the problem of evidence. *Health Informatics Journal*. **7**: 131–4.

Maynard A, Bloor K and Freemantle N (2004) Challenges for the National Institute for Clinical Excellence. *British Medical Journal*. **329**: 227–9.

Mayor S (2004a) UK body calls on UN to allow for therapeutic cloning. *British Medical Journal*. **329**: 938.

Mayor S (2004b) United Nations fails to agree on human cloning. *British Medical Journal*. **329**: 996.

Mays N (1993) Innovations in health care. In: B Davey and J Popay (eds) *Caring for Health: Dilemmas and Prospects*. The Open University, London.

McCulloch P (2004) Half full or half empty VATS? *British Medical Journal*. **329**: 1012.

McKinnon R, Worzeil K, Rotz G and Williams H (2004) *Crisis? What Crisis? A Fresh Diagnosis of Big Pharma's R&D Productivity Crunch*. Marakon Associates, London, New York.

Melzer D, Raven A, Detmer DE, Ling T and Zimmern RL (2003) *My Very Own Medicine: What must I know? Information Policy for Pharmacogenetics*. Wellcome Trust, London, Department of Public Health and Primary Care, University of Cambridge.

Mendelsohn E (1999) *Is public policy lagging behind the science?* OHE Conference on Genomics, Healthcare and Public Policy. Office of Health Economics, London, pp. 64–93.

Nelkin D (1992) The social power of genetic information. In: D Kevles and L Hood (eds) *The Code of Codes, Scientific and Social Issues in Human Genome Project*. Harvard University Press, Cambridge, MA.

Newhouse JP (1992) Medical Care Costs: How Much Welfare Loss? *Journal of Economic Perspectives*. **6**(3): 3–21.

NIH (2002) *Stem Cell Information*. http://stemcells.nih.gov/index.asp;. Accessed: 24 May 2004.

NIH (2005) *HIH Roadmap. Accelerating medical discovery to improve health.* http://nihroadmap.nih.gov. Accessed: 4 April 2005.

Norris AC (2001) *Essentials of Telemedicine and Telecare.* Wiley, Chichester, West Sussex.

Packer C (2004) *Horizon scanning for new & emerging health technologies.* National Horizon Scanning Centre, Birmingham.

Peckham M (2000a) Innovation and the future of health services. In: *A Model for Health: Innovation and the Future of Health Services.* The Nuffield Trust, London, pp. 119–43.

Peckham M (2000b) *A Model for Health: Innovation and the Future of Health Services.* The Nuffield Trust, London.

Pemberton J, Buehring A, Stonehouse G, Simpson L and Purves I (2003) Issues and trends in computerisation within UK primary health care. *Logistics Information Management.* **16**(3/4): 181–90.

Personal MD (1999a) *Artificial Fingers Created Using Cow Cells.* http://www.personalmd.com/news/a1999062911.shtml. Accessed: 1 March 2004.

Personal MD (1999b) *Telemedicine Helps Experts Diagnose Skin Cancer.* http://www.personalmd.com/news/a1999062912.shtml. Accessed: 4 April 2005.

Poole-Wilson P (1998) The heart and circulation. In: M Marinker and M Peckham (eds) *Clinical Futures.* BMJ Publications, London.

Poulter NR (2004) NICE and BHS guidelines on hypertension differ importantly. *British Medical Journal.* **329**: 1289.

Prasad SK, Assomull RG and Pennell DJ (2004) Recent developments in non-invasive cardiology. *British Medical Journal.* **329**: 1386–9.

Rashid A (2000) *The Impact of New Technologies on Future Primary Care.* The Nuffield Trust, London.

Ratner M and Ratner D (2003) *Nanotechnology: a gentle introduction to the next big idea.* Prentice Hall, Upper Saddle River, NJ.

Reiss T (2001) Drug discovery of the future: implications of the human genome project. *Trends in Biotechnology.* **19**(12): 496–9.

Relph K, Harrington K and Pandha H (2004) Recent developments and current status of gene therapy using viral vectors in the United Kingdom. *British Medical Journal.* **329**: 839–42.

Research for Patient Benefit Working Party (RPBWP) (2004) *Final Report.* Department of Health, London.

Rigby M (2005) Harnessing innovation in health IT – effective support and evaluated visions. In: S Dawson and C Sausman (eds) *Future Health Organisations and Systems.* Palgrave Macmillan, London.

Robert G, Gabbay J and Stevens A (1998) Which are the best information sources for identifying emerging health care technologies? An International Delphi Survey. *International Journal of Technology Assessment in Health Care.* **14**(4): 636–43.

Robins R and Metcalfe S (2004) Integrating genetics as practices of primary care. *Social Science & Medicine.* **59**: 223–33.

Royal Society and Royal Academy of Engineering (2003) *Nanotechnology: views of Scientists and Engineers.* The Royal Society, Royal Academy of Engineering, London.

Sedrakyan A, van der Meulen J, Lewsey J and Treasure T (2004a) Variation in use of video assisted thoracic surgery in the United Kingdom. *British Medical Journal.* **329**: 1011–12.

Sedrakyan A, van der Meulen J, Lewsey J and Treasure T (2004b) Video assisted thoracic surgery for treatment of pneumothorax and lung resections: systematic review of randomised clinical trials. *British Medical Journal.* **329**: 1008–10.

Sheldon T, Cullum N, Dawson D, Lankshear A, Lowson K, Watt I, West P, Wright D and Wright J (2004) What's the evidence that NICE guidance has been implemented? Results from the national evaluation using time series analysis, audit of patients' notes, and interviews. *British Medical Journal*. **329**: 999.

Snyderman R and Williams RS (2003) Prospective Medicine: The Next Health Care Transformation. *Academic Medicine*. **78**(11): 1079–84.

Standing Medical Advisory Committee (SMAC) (1997) *The path of least resistance. SMAC Sub-Group on Antimicrobial Resistance*. Department of Health, London.

Stevens A, Milne R, Lilford R and Gabbay J (1999) Keeping pace with new technologies: systems needed to identify and evaluate them. *British Medical Journal*. **319**: 1291–4.

Stevens A, Robert G and Gabbay J (1997) Identifying new health care technologies in the United Kingdom. *International Journal of Technology Assessment in Health Care*. **13**(1): 59–67.

Stix G (2002) Little big science. In: S Fritz *Understanding nanotechnology*. Warner Books, New York, pp. 6–16.

Strategy Unit (2003) *The Costs and Benefits of Genetically Modified (GM) Crops*. Strategy Unit, London.

Stratford N, Marteau T and Bobrow M (1999) Tailoring genes. In: R Jowell, J Curtice, A Park and K Thomson (eds) *British Social Attitudes, the 16th Report. Who Shares New Labour Values?* Ashgate Publishing, Aldershot, pp. 156–76.

Stratford N, Marteau T and Bobrow M (2001a) Genetic research: friend or foe? In: R Jowell, J Curtice, A Park, K Thomson, L Jarvis, C Bromley and N Stratford (eds) *British Social Attitudes: Focusing on Diversity. 17th Report*. Sage Publications, London, pp. 103–25.

Stratford N, Marteau T and Bobrow M (2001b) Genetic research: friend or foe? In: A Park, J Curtice, K Thomson, L Jarvis and C Bromley (eds) *British Social Attitudes, the 18th Report. Public Policy, Social Ties*. Sage Publications, London.

Summerton N (2004) NICE advice is not always practical. *Health Service Journal*. **114**: 22.

Sykes RB (2000) *New medicines: The practice of medicine and public policy*. The Stationery Office, London.

Tai S, Donegan C and Nazareth I (2000) Computers in general practice and the consultation: the health professionals' view. *Health Informatics Journal*. **6**: 27–31.

Tanne JH (2004) FDA approves implantable chip to access medical records. *British Medical Journal*. **329**: 1064.

The Economist (2003) *A Voyage of Discovery*. http://www.economist.com/displaystory.cfm?story_id=1647613. Accessed: 4 April 2005.

The Economist (2004a) *Fixing the drugs pipeline*. http://www.economist.com/displaystory.cfm?story_id=2477075. Accessed: 15 March 2004.

The Economist (2004b) *Up close, and personal*. http://www.economist.com/displaystory.cfm?story_id=3285968. Accessed: 4 April 2005.

The Economist (2004c) *Tooth Fairies*. http://www.economist.com/displaystory.cfm?story_id=2459140. Accessed: 2 March 2004.

The Economist (2004d) *Cloning embryos, multiplying controversies*. http://www.economist.com/agenda/displaystory.cfm?story_id=3100666. Accessed: 4 April 2005.

The Economist (2004e) Much ado about almost nothing. *The Economist*. 18 March 2004.

The Economist Technology Quarterly (2004) *Down on the pharm*. http://www.economist.com/displaystory.cfm?story_id=3171546. Accessed: 4 April 2005.

The Medical Technology Group (2004) *Making the Economic Case for Medical Technology*. The Medical Technology Group, London.

The Times (2005) Choice for the few. Ministers are running out of time to make the hospital computer work. *The Times*. 19 January 2005, 17.

Timmins N (2004) Beyond the bleak houses of the elderly. *Financial Times*. 25 May 2004, 10.

Tomlinson H (2004) Medical research 'stifled by rules'. *The Guardian*. 6 December 2004, accessed online.

US Office of Technological Assessment (1982) *Strategies for Medical Technical Assessment*. US Office of Technological Assessment, Washington, DC.

van der Lei J, Duisterhout JS, Westerhof HP, van der Does E, Cromme PVM, Boon WM and van Bemmel JH (1993) The introduction of Computer-based Patient Records in the Netherlands. *Annals of Internal Medicine*. 119(10): 1036–41.

Vats A, Tolley NS, Buttery LDK and Polak JM (2004) The stem cell in orthopaedic surgery. *The Journal of Bone & Joint Surgery*. **86-B**(2): 159–64.

Wanless D (2002) *Securing our Future Health: Taking a Long-Term View*. HM Treasury, London.

Watts G (2004) Paper prescriptions will soon be distinctly 'last season'. *British Medical Journal*. **328**: 1156.

Weinshilboum R (2003) Inheritance and drug response. *New England Journal of Medicine*. **348**: 529–37.

Wild C and Torgesen H (2000) Foresight in medicine. Lessons from three European Delphi studies. *European Journal of Public Health*. **10**: 114–19.

Williamson P (1992) From dissemination to use: Management and organisational barriers to the application of health services research findings. *Health Bulletin*. **50**(1): 78–86.

Wilsdon J and Willis R (2004) *See-through Science: Why public engagement needs to move upsteam*. Demos, London.

Wilson CB (1999) Hospitals of the future. The impact of medical technologies on the future of hospitals. *British Medical Journal*. **319**: 1287–93.

Wong G (2004) Email consultations in health care. *British Medical Journal*. **329**: 1046.

Wood S, Jones R and Geldart A (2003) *The Social and Economic Challenges of Nanotechnology*. Economic and Social Research Council, London.

Wyatt CJ and Keen J (2001) The new NHS information technology strategy. *British Medical Journal*. **322**: 1378–9.

Young T, Brailsford S, Connell C, Davies R, Harper P and Klein JH (2004) Using industrial processes to improve patient care. *British Medical Journal*. **328**: 162–4.

Ziebland S, Chapple A, Dumelow C, Evans J, Prinjha S and Rozmovits L (2004) How the internet affects patients' experience of cancer: a qualitative study. *British Medical Journal*. **328**: 564–7.

Zimmern RL and Cook C (2000) *The Nuffield Trust Genetics Scenario Project: genetics and health policy issues for genetic science and their implications for health and health services*. Nuffield Trust, London.

Chapter 8

What will health cost?

Graham Lister and Ray Robinson

While the production of health is the primary objective of all healthcare systems, these systems are not the only (or arguably, the most important) determinants of health. According to WHO's definition (1946), 'Health is a complete state of physical, mental and social wellbeing and not merely the absence of disease or infirmity'. This definition highlights the fact that health, as an output, is determined by a range of inputs including environmental factors, employment, public health legislation, social care, action to support self-care, wellness and lifestyle choices and investment in global health. In this chapter, a production function view of health is taken and broad indicative cost estimates are provided for the main inputs to health.

The chapter considers how these costs are likely to change and how they are to be met in 2020 – namely, by whom and how they are to be paid – and the balance between them in terms of, *inter alia*, programme expenditures and the combination of public/private spending. It concludes that the costs of poor health, which fall on individuals, carers, local and central government and employers, are of a similar magnitude to healthcare costs and are likely to increase significantly over the next 15 years. The 'fully engaged' scenario as called for in the Wanless report (2004) will require an extension of the sources of funding for health and care, as well as actions to promote informed engagement with health by all sectors of society.

Central taxation is expected to remain the basis for funding National Health Service (NHS) services, although other forms of funding will be of increasing importance for self-care and long-term care of people with complex physical, mental and social care needs. These conditions are seen as the defining challenges for future health and care funding. This perspective provides a wider context to the question of whether tax funding for the NHS will be sustainable over the next 15 years. Central taxation is likely to remain the primary source of funding for the NHS but it will be necessary to control healthcare costs by better commissioning and a clearer definition of patient rights.

The role of the Department of Health (DH) is expected to change, from the targeting and direction of healthcare provision, to the stewardship of health commissioning, provision and regulation. In the future, the NHS could be characterised as a tax-funded system guaranteeing access to cost-effective treatment choices. These would be commissioned by local health organisations from a network of community, voluntary and privately-owned health and social care organisations, all competing to attract patients on the basis of service and quality. More private providers will be encouraged to participate in the NHS-funded marketplace.

Since the NHS in other home countries is not following this path, whether it continues as a vertically-managed public sector system outside England will depend upon the success or failure of the NHS in England, particularly when the rate of increase in health funding slows. An equally important task for home country departments of health will be to provide leadership for health nationally, while supporting local leadership and action for health by all sectors of society. A new Health of the People Act and a range of measures to support wider engagement with health are proposed.

Healthcare

The most authoritative forecast of the need for healthcare funding is provided by the *Wanless Review*. This is based on a calculation of the increases required to improve quality standards to meet the National Service Frameworks, and adjusted for changes in demographic factors and of other trends under three different scenarios for the future of health (Wanless, 2002).

The review was accepted by the government as the basis for NHS funding increases over the next four years. Between 2002/03 and 2007/08, NHS funding is set to increase by an average of 7.4% per annum in real terms. After 2008, the rate of increase in NHS expenditure required was assumed to reduce significantly to between 4.3 and 3.2% per annum in real terms, about the rate of increase from 1954 to 2000. NHS expenditure is projected to rise from £68 billion in 2002/03 to between £154 and £184 billion in 2022/23 in real terms (that is after consumer price inflation).

The *Wanless Review* suggests that 'the lower' scenario for NHS costs could be achieved by the full engagement of society in responsible health choices. This 'fully engaged' scenario represents the ideal of a transformation in attitudes to health, which is assumed to lead to greater savings than the marginal benefits of individual public health measures as measured by Ableson (2003). It is also possible that attitudes to health will not change and a 'higher cost' scenario will apply.

The review states that taxation is the most efficient and equitable basis for funding the NHS and proposes no changes. The 'fully engaged' scenario is said to be affordable to the state and likely to be comparable to, or lower than, spending in competitor countries (Lister, 2005). Wanless has stated on a number of occasions that he doubts the feasibility of funding the higher range scenarios for health costs.

Underlying cost drivers identified in the 2000 *Policy Futures for UK Health* report (Dargie, 2000) include:

- rising expectations of quality and choice as standards of living increase
- the need to improve services to ethnic minority communities
- and technological developments, particularly genetics and stem cell research.

These trends, which were not fully considered by Wanless, are likely to lead to pressure to increase NHS spending at 4 to 5% per annum for the following ten years (Lister, 2005). It is therefore important to ask whether the funding and spending regime for the NHS will be robust enough to control costs and achieve efficiency savings once the period of rapid increases in funding ends.

The mechanisms for directing healthcare spending within the NHS in England are currently in transition. Primary Care Trusts (PCTs) are allocated and control 81% of NHS expenditure, as commissioners through contracts defined by the PCTs or GP practices with NHS Trusts and other healthcare providers. The 302 PCTs managed average commissioning budgets of £150 million in 2002/03. The remaining 19% is allocated directly by the DH through central purchasing and commissioning arrangements. The performance of all Trusts is monitored by 28 Strategic

Health Authorities on the basis of agreements and targets reflecting government commitments set out in the NHS Plan and guidance from the National Institute for Clinical Excellence (NICE) and other bodies. Although this centrally-driven performance management system, based on targets and sanctions, has been the subject of much criticism, it has driven a remarkable improvement in health service delivery (DH, 2004a).

Foundation Trusts achieve independence by performing well and gaining high ratings from the Healthcare Commission. They must also demonstrate sound management and governance, which includes the engagement of patients and staff as members and owners of the Trust. They are then able to raise funds and negotiate agreements with PCTs and others for the provision of health services, free of the performance management regime operated by Strategic Health Authorities. In February 2005, there were 20 authorised Foundation Trusts and a further 20 applicants. It is envisaged that in 15 years time virtually all NHS services in England will be provided by a combination of such community enterprises and privately-owned healthcare providers.

At the same time a standard system of tariffs is being introduced for Health Resource Groups (HRGs). It will establish case-mix adjusted cost and volume contracts with the aim of covering virtually all HRGs by 2006 (DH, 2004b). This will mean that providers will compete at the same price level to attract patients, advised by GPs, on the grounds of patient service and quality. The regulation regime for Foundation Trusts, undertaken by a new agency called Monitor, is designed to ensure that they comply with their Terms of Authorisation and avoid undue risks. This should prevent them from 'cherry picking' only the most profitable services or offering unproven services. However, Foundation Trusts will be able to raise private finance, diversify and grow by taking on new health services and run the risk of insolvency, if politicians are prepared to let this happen. They will have an incentive to increase the services they offer, while PCTs will need to control costs by commissioning a defined package of cost-effective services reflecting health needs.

Thus, in the critical period when public investment in health slows down, NHS performance will be determined by regulated market competition, with PCTs commissioning services from a horizontal network of community and privately-owned providers. This strategy is crucially dependent upon the quality of the commissioning function undertaken by PCTs. There is a need to provide greater support for this function and to clarify patient entitlement (or rights) under the NHS.

The other home countries have not adopted this reform path. Their NHS services are directed by home country departments of health, with performance and commissioning managed by Health Boards. There are four Health Boards in Northern Ireland, 15 in Scotland and 22 in Wales. They contract with publicly-owned NHS Trusts which provide services. These can be described as vertical public sector structures.

Private sector spend on healthcare (excluding long-term residential care) in 2002 was £14 billion. It has risen continuously since 1987 and seems likely to continue to rise. In total, private payments account for 17% of UK healthcare compared with an average of 25% across the EU (Social Market Foundation, 2003). Forms of private spending include:

- health insurance
- cash plans
- dental plans

- critical illness insurance
- income protection and long-term care insurance
- co-payment
- direct payment.

Private spending on healthcare is, however, likely to remain a supplement rather than a substitute for public spending (Mossialos and Thomson, 2004).

Personal care

In 2000, two-thirds of NHS hospital beds were used by people aged over 65. Many of these patients suffer from chronic diseases or long-term conditions, requiring a combination of health and personal care. While the onset of infirmity is being delayed in many countries, years of poor health are not decreasing (Wiener *et al.*, 1994). Men in the UK have an average life expectancy of 76 years with nine years of poor health, while women have an average life expectancy of 80 years and 12 years of poor health (ONS, 2004a).

Older people comprise half of those with impairments and disabilities, often requiring long-term care, the total cost of which was £10.5 billion in 1999/2000 (DH, 2000a). The boundary between health and personal care is increasingly blurred. Many initiatives are underway aimed at better management of long-term chronic conditions. The 'Evercare' model brought to England from the US, for example, combines a more active primary care 'Community Matron' nursing role with coordinated care and intervention to reduce the need for hospital admission (DH, 2004c).

In 1999, the Sutherland Commission called for long-term care costs to be split between personal care, living and housing costs (1999). It argued for personal care costs to be assessed on the basis of need and paid for by general taxation, while living and housing costs were to be subject to co-payment according to means. The government responded that steps would be taken to provide free NHS nursing care but free personal care would be too expensive in England.

In Scotland, free home personal care was introduced in 2002, together with an allowance to pay for personal and nursing care for people in long-term care homes. It was estimated that this provision would cost £1.5 billion (Machin and McShane, 2001), but demand increased and it is now estimated that costs will rise by a further £1 billion over the next 15 years (BBC, 2004). The Welsh Assembly, like Northern Ireland, followed the English model (Woodhouse, 2000).

Personal and nursing care, provided by the NHS and local authorities, is a small percentage of total care. Informal care provided by spouses or others is between eight and ten times greater for those under 75; for those over 75 this ratio drops to 3.7 because relatives are often no longer able to assist (Machin and McShane, 2001). By 2020, the number of UK residents dependent upon informal care could increase from 2.5 million to 4 million, and the number of people over 75 will increase by more than 20%. Currently there are 16 million carers, the value of whose work has been estimated at £57.4 billion a year (Carers UK, 2002).

Projections of the cost of long-term care for the elderly by Wittenberg *et al.* (2002a) suggest that expenditure could rise from 1.37% to between 1.5 and 1.8% of GDP by 2020. Currently, 66% of long-term care is publicly funded, but with free personal care this could increase to 79%.

The funding of long-term care is a major challenge, not just for the next 15 years but for the next 50 years, since by 2051 it is estimated that care spending will need to triple in real terms (Wittenberg *et al.*, 2002b). While it can be argued that the current balance of tax and insurance funding could cope with this level of increase there is a need for a serious debate about dedicated forms of social insurance or private insurance to establish a stable and equitable basis for long-term care funding. This raises issues of cross-generational equity, since it may require those in work to fund the increasing burden of care for those beyond working age or to increase their pension or insurance provision to provide for their own long-term care needs. Inheritance may be affected by the use of housing equity to fund care. It has been suggested that pension funds could be linked to long-term health and care invest-ment as one response to this problem. It is also important to note that in the next 15 years the dependency ratio (those outside working age as a ratio of those of working age) will be relatively stable as the age of retirement for women is extended, but beyond 2020 there will be a sharp increase in this ratio.

Public health

Resources devoted to public health include 1331 consultants and specialists in public health in the UK, just over half of whom are employed in the NHS, a quarter in universities, a sixth in Communicable Disease Control, with others employed by government, including Regional Administrative Offices, and the private sector (Perlman and Gray, 2004). The front line for public health information, advice and monitoring is provided by multi-professional primary care teams, including GPs, practice nurses, and health visitors who are public health nurses (Gray, 1995).

The DH also funds public health observatories at Regional Administrative office levels in England and advertising campaigns contracted to non-governmental organisations. The most recent government health White Paper *Choosing Health: making healthy choices easier* (DH, 2004d) proposes a new taskforce with responsi-bility for public health information, intelligence and social marketing for health. A broad estimate based on discussion with Professor Hunter, President of the UK Public Health Association, is that the NHS and DH spend about £600 million on public health functions.

Local Authority Environmental Health departments – whose role is to minimise risks to public health arising from air and water pollution, poor hygiene in restaurants and shops and pests – play an important role in the protection of health and addressing the broader determinants of health, as noted by Burke *et al.* (2002). There are also Building Control Officers, concerned with the safety of buildings and construction, Trading Standards Officers, who, as Butterworth (2003) notes, are also important resources for public health, and 74 local authorities that operate Port Health Services. A broad estimate by the authors is that local government spends £500 million on public health functions.

National agencies engaged in public health include the Health Protection Agency – which monitors and coordinates response to risks arising from infectious diseases, radiation, chemical and biochemical hazards and poisons, the Food Standards Agency, the Health and Safety Executive and the Environment Agency. The total budget of these agencies in 2003/04 was £1.5 billion.

Responsibility for and expenditure on public health functions is split between the NHS, local authorities and national agencies. Total expenditure is in the region of

£2.5 billion. *Choosing Health* suggests that total expenditure on public health and self-care will be increased by £1 billion over the next five years (DH, 2004d).

Self-care and wellness

Self-care is the predominant mode of treatment for minor illnesses. Coulter and Magee (2003) report that in the UK, 55% of survey respondents reported that in case of minor illness they would self-care (26% said they would visit the doctor, 17% said they would take no action). The Proprietary Association of Great Britain report a survey that showed that in cases of minor illnesses, 46% were untreated, 9% used home remedies, 26% used over-the-counter medicines bought for the purpose, 14% used medicines found in the home and only 10% said they visited the doctor (Bell, 2003). The market for self-medication and food supplements was valued at £1.97 billion in 2002 (Proprietary Association of Great Britain, 2003).

The decision to allow the sale of Simvastatin without prescription is notable because it recognises the role of pharmacists as partners with the NHS in delivering preventive healthcare (DH, 2003a). Simvastatin prescription by pharmacists involves continuous monitoring of cholesterol levels and advice on diet and lifestyle, a role which in the past has been the prerogative of GPs and practice nurses. Many GPs find this anomalous, arguing that such treatment requires a wider range of tests and can lead to complications, that pharmacists have a commercial interest in sales and that it is wrong to provide treatment on the basis of ability to pay. However, this may be seen as a radical new model for self-care, promoted by advertising, chosen and paid for by the customer and favouring those who are well informed and can afford to pay.

Self-care is recognised as central to chronic physical and mental illness. The Expert Patient Programme has proved to be remarkably successful in empowering patients to develop coping strategies to address chronic health, social and personal needs. It also demonstrates the need to support self-care and the important role that voluntary sector organisations, such as patient groups, can play in articulating and meeting this need (Johnson, 2004). It provides an example of health and care as co-created goods produced by patients, community and health services (Cottam and Leadbeater, 2004).

The willingness of the public to engage with their health and wellness is shown by the consumption of health products and services. The UK market for gyms and health clubs reached £1.6 billion in 2001 with 18% of adults claiming to attend. Local authorities provided 37% of this market. The market is focused on adults under the age of 45 with higher levels of income (Hasler and Cooney, 2002). The total UK market for sport and fitness-related products, including sports equipment and clothing, is estimated at £6.3 billion (FCO, 1999).

To improve access to sport and activity for disadvantaged groups, a programme was initiated in 1999 to provide Healthy Living Centres. These would offer a range of health advice and support, including physical activity and gym provision to 20% of the population in greatest need. The programme covers all home countries and is funded by £300 million Lottery grants, managed by the New Opportunities Fund. Community sports and physical activity in England are also supported by Sports England and the Big Lottery Fund, who are investing £108 million in initiatives with a special focus on areas of multiple deprivation (DH, 2004e). In December 2004, a further initiative was announced to combat obesity in children by providing two hours of sport and physical education in school hours, as well as access to a further two hours of sport outside the curriculum. This is to be supported by additional expenditure of £459 million, bringing total spending to £1.5 billion in the period 2003–08 (DCMS, 2004).

The market for reduced fat and reduced calorie food reached £5.2 billion in 2000 and grew by 17.4% between 2001 and 2003 (Mintel International Group Ltd, 2003). Over the next 15 years, the public will be willing to engage with their health and pay for health products, although further measures will be required to inform their choices and to improve access for low income groups.

Local engagement in wellness must respond to and reflect community structures and leadership. The Local Government Act 2000 gave local authorities a new duty to prepare community strategies for local economic, social and environmental wellbeing (Office of the Deputy Prime Minister, 2003). This draws from the experience of Health Action Zones (HAZs) in England, which started work in 1998, funded by £270 million government grants to build partnerships between health agencies, local authorities, voluntary and private sector organisations. These developed into Local Strategic Partnerships (LSPs) drawing on a range of resources and commitments for health and wellbeing (DH, 2004e). While neither HAZs nor LSPs have yet proved to be universally successful, *Choosing Health* will attempt to build on best practice in the engagement of individuals and communities in health (DH, 2004d). Poverty is the single clearest cause of ill health and lack of access to health services, products and information (LGA *et al.*, 2004). Local engagement is therefore focused on disadvantaged individuals and groups. The importance of the arts to mental health and wellbeing is becoming increasingly evident. The Arts Council is currently producing a national strategy for arts and health, which may lead to systematic funding (Staricoff, 2004).

Support for self-care is provided by NHS Direct nurse-operated telephone call centres and online services, which will shortly include a new range of Health Direct Services providing advice on health choices (DH, 2004f). In December 2004, a Digital Interactive Television form of NHS Direct was launched on a satellite television channel, providing access to some 3000 Internet pages of health information and advice and video clips on a range of health topics (DH, 2004g). This is only the first step towards the provision of a range of television-based services, which can be tailored to support the self-care needs of local groups and individuals. It will also be important in terms of enabling people to maintain their own guides to personal health and wellness, using the 'Healthspace' facility to maintain their own electronic personal health plan. There is also a range of commercially-funded television channels featuring health and wellness. It is estimated that the full cost of all such services could amount to £300 to £500 million.

Further positive measures to support healthy behaviour are proposed in *Choosing Health* (DH, 2004d). These include the development of community champions for health, steps to promote corporate social responsibility for health, provision of personal trainers to help individuals and families to address their health issues and adopt healthy practices. The White Paper also proposes a system of 'Traffic Lights' markings, operated by the Food Standards Agency to indicate foods that are healthy, need to be eaten in moderation or are unhealthy. In support of these and other measures to improve healthy choices, the government is committed to increasing expenditure by £1 billion.

Lifestyle factors

Many of the costs of ill health may be attributed to lifestyle factors, which in some cases are also a source of tax revenues, as noted below:

- the costs of tobacco-related illness to the NHS are estimated at £1.5 billion per year; tobacco taxes raised £8 billion in 2002/03 (ASH, 2004)
- the direct cost of alcohol to the NHS is estimated at £200 million. The total cost of alcohol-related sickness, absence, injury and crime is estimated at £3.3 billion; taxes on alcohol raised £5 billion in 2002/03 (Alcohol Concern, 2000)
- obesity is estimated to result in costs to the economy of £3.3 to 3.7 billion. Obesity and overweight results in costs of £6.6 to £7.4 billion (House of Commons Health Committee, 2004)
- it is estimated that Class A illegal drug use costs society between £10 billion and £17.4 billion per year (HDA, 2003).

There are some fields in which taxation can be used as a means of reflecting the externality costs imposed by unhealthy consumption. VAT rates and excise duty are applied to make healthy products and activities cheaper than unhealthy choices. While retail food in general bears no VAT, for example, certain products such as ice cream, crisps, salted nuts, confectionary and some other savoury snacks are subject to VAT, and alcohol and cigarettes also bear excise duty. Positive subsidy is also used to support healthy behaviour, for example health and fitness sessions prescribed by some GPs at reduced cost or free and the provision of free fruit at schools, funded by £42 million from Lottery sources, have had substantial health benefits (DH, 2001).

Choosing Health also proposes measures to ban smoking in public premises, such as restaurants and bars serving food, where employees or other customers may be subject to secondary smoking harm (DH, 2004d). This step reflects the success of action taken in Ireland and proposals for a more stringent ban on smoking in Scotland.

Health and work

Ill health is a major cost to industry and work is a major cause of ill health. Total absence from work in 2002/03 resulted in 176 million lost working days, costing industry £11.6 billion. It is estimated that some 15% of these absences were not related to sickness, so the total cost of sickness was £10 billion. Absences increased from 2001–02 when 166 million days were lost (CBI, 2004).

Another survey shows that 32.9 million days lost due to illness were caused or made worse by work (ONS, 2002). The main illnesses caused by or related to work were stress, depression or anxiety, which accounted for 13.5 million days off work, and musculoskeletal disorders, which accounted for 12.3 million lost working days. In total, 2.3 million illnesses were said to have been caused by or made worse by current or past work.

The CBI survey quoted above shows that the higher levels of sickness and absenteeism were consistently recorded by large organisations and the public sector, as compared to small private sector companies. *Choosing Health* (DH, 2004d) has recognised the importance of ensuring that the NHS takes measures to make itself an exemplary organisation, by providing positive health programmes for its staff and managing sickness and absenteeism.

Sickness and incapacity are also major factors in unemployment: in 2003, some 2.7 million unemployed adults claimed sickness-related benefits. The diversion of some people from unemployment to incapacity benefits distorts the underlying trend in unemployment by up to one million (Beatty and Fothergill, 2004; Bell and Smith, 2004). The total cost to the public sector of disability benefit is £6 billion. The recent consultative paper on this topic is called *Pathways to Work: helping people into employment* (DWP, 2005). It proposes that, from 2008, benefits paid to those with severe incapacity should be increased. At the same time, those assessed with lesser levels of incapacity who could benefit from work will have benefits reduced to the level of job seeker's allowances unless they take steps to find employment.

European countries that achieve high levels of investment in public health – The Netherlands, Sweden and Finland – include substantial occupational health schemes to which all employers are obliged to contribute (CREDES, 2002). In the US, it is estimated that 93% of companies offer health promotion and management (Kickbusch and Payne, 2003). By contrast, although some employers provide a range of positive health programmes, UK employer contribution to public health is mostly limited to health and safety measures (Health and Safety Commission, 1999). *Choosing Health* (DH, 2004d) notes the initiative by the Health and Safety Executive called *Constructing Better Health*. This is an occupational health support pilot programme for the construction industry, jointly funded by industry and government. It provides a range of health screening and positive health support elements, and could lead to schemes for other industries. Dr Robson, Chair of the British Medical Association (BMA) Occupational Health Committee, has called for further investment in occupational health (Robson, 2004).

Some industries already incur substantial costs relating to health and environmental protection. The Water Research Centre estimates that meeting the 1991 EU nitrates directive will cost the UK some £4 billion (DEFRA, 2003), for example, while the cost of regulations regarding the control of asbestos at work was estimated at £4.8 billion (Gooday, 2000), and the cost impact of the BSE crisis was estimated at £3.7 billion (Phillips *et al.*, 2000). This suggests a total annualised cost for health and environmental externalities of at least £3 billion.

These cases are considered by specially-constituted inquiries. In each case consultation leads to a decision to allocate costs between government, industry and the consumer, however, there is no mechanism for ensuring consistency in such judgements or for looking ahead at future potential risks.

The cost of road traffic accidents is estimated at £10.9 billion (based on actual costs and the amount people would be prepared to pay to avoid accidents). Expenditure on road safety measures is estimated at £2.2 billion per year, of which £1.2 billion is attributable to personal and business expenditure (PACTS, 2000). The provision of advanced train protection systems is estimated to cost £6 billion over an unspecified period (Uff and Cullen, 2001). In 1998, road traffic accidents were responsible for 3421 deaths and 325 000 injuries, while there were 19 deaths and 2710 injuries attributed to rail accidents.

Global health

As Brundtland explained, investment in health as a global public good is in our own interest: 'With globalisation, a single microbial sea washes all of humankind. There are no health sanctuaries' (Brundtland, 2000). In 2003/04, the UK invested some

£316 million in bilateral aid for health and a further £100–120 million through multilateral agencies (Lister, 2005). In addition there were expenditures of one to two million pounds by the Health Protection Agency on international collaboration and disease surveillance. While all UK aid is ostensibly devoted to alleviating poverty and promoting sustainable development, investment in global health also serves to protect the long-term health and security of the UK population. It has been suggested that the UN target of devoting 0.7% of GDP to official development aid should be supplemented by a further target for investment in global public goods such as health, from which all benefit and none can be excluded (Kickbusch and Payne, 2004).

Funding health and healthcare

UK National Accounts for Health (ONS, 2004b) show total expenditures in 2002 of £80.6 billion (7.7% of GDP) from government, the private sector, households and charities for the healthcare purposes of:

- promoting health and preventing disease
- curing illness and reducing premature mortality
- caring for persons affected by chronic illness who require nursing care
- caring for people with health-related impairment, disability, and handicaps who require nursing care
- assisting patients to die with dignity
- providing and administering public health
- providing and administering health programmes, health insurance and other funding arrangements.

It has not been possible to accurately assess all other costs of poor health to society, but the figures noted in the preceding sections, excluding those costs noted above and informal care, amount to some £35 billion. If the cost of informal care is taken into account, this sum would increase to approximately £90 billion. Moreover, these broader costs of health are likely to grow over the next 15 years, since in many cases they depend upon ageing and lifestyle factors that are difficult to change. By 2020, the UK may face 11.4% of GDP in healthcare costs as projected by Wanless. The broader costs of health and wellness could total a similar amount, constituting in total over 20% of GDP in costs to individuals, employers, charities, local authorities and the NHS. This would follow trends in the US where the 'wellness' market is estimated to have reached $200 billion and is projected to grow to $1 trillion over the next ten years, comparable to healthcare (Pilzer, 2002).

It would be helpful to extend the development of national health accounts, which follow OECD guidelines, to encompass the full cost of ill health to society (Lister *et al.*, in press). Health status could be used as an indicator of future health liabilities and investments in actions to promote future health. It would also be possible to evaluate health impacts on and from the rest of the world, as is done in the National Environmental Accounts, to account for health as a global public good (ONS, 2004c).

While health systems in different countries are characterised as either social insurance, tax-funded or private insurance based, in practice health costs are supported by a combination of funding sources as discussed below. The sources of funding for European healthcare systems have been examined by Mossialos *et al.* (2002) and were reviewed by the Chancellor of the Exchequer in a speech to the Social Market Foundation (Brown, 2002).

Central taxation

Central taxation currently funds 84% of NHS provision and NHS expenditure is 83% of total healthcare funding (CREDES, 2002). Wanless (2002) states that taxation should remain the basis for funding the NHS and this view is supported by a range of other commentators (Mossialos and Le Grand, 1999; Saltman and Figueras, 1998) who suggest that tax remains the most efficient method of tax collection, the most effective way of controlling expenditure and the most equitable way of sharing health risks.

A different perspective is provided by Harrison and Moran (2000), who note that 'free' healthcare creates a moral hazard for patients to overuse health services and to disregard personal responsibility for their health and that of their families. They argue that tax-funded services fail to provide incentives that encourage providers to treat patients with dignity and personal attention.

To counter these moral hazards, steps have been taken by successive govern-ments to reinforce individual rights and responsibility for health and responsible use of services, see for example *Patient's Charter* (DH, 1996). Current policy is to ensure that patient standards are not only surveyed and monitored but are underpinned by patient choice. By December 2005, all patients will be able to choose between four or five providers of elective care, which should include NHS and Foundation Trusts, Independent Sector Hospitals, NHS and Independent Sector Treatment Centres or extended Primary Care Treatment Services (DH, 2004f).

It has also been argued that public payment systems lead to a moral hazard for health suppliers to induce demand or to focus on the most lucrative services. Although this argument has diminished in the UK since the introduction of the purchaser/provider structure in 1991, it is still important to ensure that there is a balance between the powers of purchasers and providers (Donaldson and Gerard, 1989).

As in the UK, Canada has many pundits who claim that public funding will be unsustainable in the future and that greater reliance will need to be placed on private finance. Robert Evans argues that this claim cannot be supported by the empirical evidence and that those who make it are really supporting a pro-rich redistribution of payments and benefits, through a movement to private funding (Evans, 2002; 2005). Reinhardt (Reinhardt, 2001) argues that sustainability is not really about expenditure trends at all, but is a moral issue – a debate about what members of society owe each other.

Local authority funding

Local authority funding for long-term care and aspects of public health is estimated at £7.1 billion – 9% of total healthcare costs (CREDES, 2002). Funding through local authorities (derived from local and central taxes) provides a way of matching services to local preferences and requirements, with broadly based democratic involvement. This may mean that clinical input to decision making is reduced and specialist medical needs may be overlooked.

In relation to public health, the requirement to involve local people and to match actions to local needs may create benefits that offset such disadvantages. Since local authorities are responsible for a significant element of current public health expenditures and also control powers relating to economic and social development, increasing their capabilities in relation to other aspects of public engagement with health could bring greater local focus and coordination.

As already noted, for an increasing number of people the boundary between health and personal care is difficult to define. There are dangers of either applying inappropriate medical models to such people or subjecting them to a multiplicity of ill-connected services provided by different agencies. Turning Point claims that £7.83 billion is wasted each year by the gap between health and social care services in England (Turning Point, 2004). One solution is to establish a holistic view of social, psychological and medical needs for people with complex requirements and to fund whole packages of service to address such needs. This requires local authorities and PCTs to combine their funding and commissioning functions through Local Strategic Partnerships, but differences in funding mechanisms, lack of alignment of boundaries and differences in professional approaches pose problems. The Local Government Association, the UK Public Health Association and the National Health Confederation have recently proposed that boundaries should be aligned (2004). This could lead to the development of further Care Trusts, combining physical and mental health and social care (there are currently eight in England).

Health and social care are aligned through integrated health and social care boards in Northern Ireland, Community Health Partnerships in Scotland and local partnerships between health and social care agencies in Wales. In Wales, the review of health and social care advised by Wanless (2003) was critical of the performance of the system in delivering preventive care and saw this as one cause of the poor value for money achieved by health and care expenditure. The Welsh Assembly is therefore giving particular attention to this issue.

There is a case for funding long-term health and social care for people assessed as having multiple needs through a form of voucher or patient-held budget. This is standard practice in The Netherlands and ensures that these patients take the lead in choosing care programmes that meet their specific needs, are well-integrated and take account of informal care. In Germany, patients are offered the choice of a package of care or a lower cost payment to enable them to finance their own care (Wittenberg et al., 2002b). This does not suit all patients but could be a powerful force to bring much-needed reform to care services and should be studied for application in this country.

Social insurance funding

Social insurance funding accounted for 11% of total healthcare and 13% of NHS funding in 2000 (CREDES, 2002). In 2002, employer and employee contributions were increased as a way of meeting future health costs (Chancellor of the Exchequer, 2002). National Insurance is not linked to health service provision as a contributory right, however, and can therefore be regarded as simply another source of general taxation. While it would be possible to increase total National Insurance premiums to the level required to fund the NHS, this would have a number of serious disadvantages. It would increase employment costs and would introduce economic instability because demand for health services tends to rise as employment declines (Acheson, 1998).

Proposals for the evolution of various forms of social health insurance for the NHS have been put forward by the Health Policy Consensus Group including giving patients choice of the PCT they would contract with through a voucher scheme, PCTs becoming consumer mutuals owned by their patients, or PCTs becoming provider-led healthcare maintenance organisations (Bosanquet *et al.*, 2003).

Other employer payments

Other employer payments are used in some countries to provide occupational health services or to pay a tax to enable these services to be provided. Current employer contributions to the NHS through National Insurance have been estimated at £5 per employee per week (Brown, 2002). Over the next 15 years, ways of improving occupational health in the UK may include encouragement and championing of best practice and possibly a levy similar to the funding of industrial training, which when first introduced, recognised existing good practice and required large employers to contribute to industry-based schemes.

Product or 'sin' taxes

Taxes on items contributing to ill health are used by many countries to fund aspects of public health. In the UK, while there are taxes on tobacco, alcohol, gambling and some fast food products, there has been no link to health funding until 2002, when an additional tax on tobacco producing revenues of £300 million was introduced specifically as hypothecated tax for health purposes (Chancellor of the Exchequer, 2002).

One problem with such taxes is that, in many cases, the relationship between causes of ill health and outcomes is complex, long-term and uncertain. For example, asthma, allergies, obesity and hyperactivity in children are all rising rapidly but it is difficult to identify single causes. Thus, Monaghan *et al.* (2003) propose a process:

- where a product, or practice, is believed to contribute to a potential health problem, a community group or public health agency would make a *prima facie* case for review
- if accepted the vendor or producer would be required to pay a surcharge, which in aggregate would pay for the research, and to indicate that the product was under review, using the 'traffic lights' system
- as an alternative, producers may prefer to take steps to avoid being subject to review by voluntary compliance (such as reducing salt, sugar or fat levels)
- research would then indicate evidence-based regulatory action, which could include banning the product or service, limiting advertising and displaying a warning using the 'traffic lights', for example, stating how many packets of a product would exceed the maximum recommended level of salt, or the application of VAT or duty.

This proposal is intended to have a threefold effect: to reduce the consumption of harmful products, raise revenues reflecting the full costs to society of the ill health caused and signal health issues so that producers and consumers will address them.

Private payment and insurance

Private payment and insurance accounts for 17% of total healthcare spending (£14 billion) and 34% of expenditure on long-term care (£4 billion).

The Social Market Foundation suggests that a privately-financed sector is an important and growing part of overall health spending in the UK. It allows choice, provides a safety valve for those whom the NHS has failed and provides for innovation in responding to patients. They do not propose any form of subsidy to the private sector (Social Market Foundation, 2003).

Moral hazards that apply to private insurance include both over-consumption by patients, over-treatment by health providers and adverse selection by insurers. HIV/AIDS and the availability of genetic information have raised the need to regulate health insurance so that there is no adverse selection on such grounds. Health insurers can, however, still target lower risk groups, such as people of working age. Tuohy *et al.* (2004), suggest that one reason why the provision of private healthcare in the UK has not resulted in a fall in NHS waiting times is because it is in clinicians' interests to encourage higher levels of private treatment.

Long-term care requires a combination of public and private insurance and payment (Wiener *et al.*, 1994). Options being explored to increase private insurance funding of long-term care in the UK include development of a market for long-term care insurance and measures based on releasing a stake in people's homes. These schemes are reported by the Treasury to have had limited take-up (2001). It is essential to find a long-term solution that is affordable and fair, to rich and poor and between generations. A further study of this issue is required.

Co-payment funding

Co-payments in the UK are limited to prescription medicines (but 80% are exempt), adult dentistry and some services in hospitals (parking, televisions and amenity beds). Co-payment makes up less than 5% of NHS funding (it is much higher in the private sector) and 11% of total health costs (Robinson, 2002). It can provide incentives for more responsible use of health services. In Sweden, for example, patients pay a limited fee to visit their doctor and as a consequence Sweden has the lowest rate of GP contact in Europe and a much higher rate of contact with public health nurses (CREDES, 2002). Research evidence indicates, however, that co-payment can be both inefficient and inequitable, leading to a less than optimal use of services, particularly by disadvantaged groups. The Chancellor of the Exchequer has expressed his opinion that co-payment can result in delayed primary care treatment and higher long-term health costs (Brown, 2002).

Changing circumstances, however, may suggest that there is a case for examining co-payment in the broader context of health. It would seem possible to apply co-payment to choices which do not affect the quality of health or health services. There is no reason, for example, why the ingredient costs of patients' meals should be lower than those served in prisons. Patients' choices resulting in additional costs to the NHS could be surcharged, for example non-attendance at appointments has been estimated to cost the NHS £300 million per annum (Hamilton *et al.*, 1999). It is timely to re-examine charges for prescription medicines, holiday vaccination, travel and other items to ensure that they do not have negative effects for health or equity. The Welsh Assembly and Scottish Parliament are already committed to eliminating prescription charges (Citizens Advice Bureau, 2001).

Capital funding

Capital funding of the NHS in England is dominated by public–private partnership investment. Investment in capital stock in the NHS in the form of buildings is currently estimated at £3.3 billion per annum, 70% of which is provided from private sources (DH, 2002a).

In 2001, there were 64 major public–private partnership construction schemes in progress with a total capital cost of £8.5 billion. A further 29 new hospital schemes were announced in that year (DH, 2002b). In addition, the NHS Plan (DH, 2000b) proposed 20 new Diagnosis and Treatment Centres funded by public–private partnership and eight more centres have since been proposed (DH, 2004h). In 2003 the Local Investment Finance Trust scheme was introduced for the development of primary and community care facilities, again by public–private partnership (DH, 2004i). The NHS Information Infrastructure (NHSII) project was announced in 2004, financed by private sector resources at a total cost of £6.2 billion. In total, the Treasury estimate that 28.4% of capital investment for the NHS in 2003/04 will be from public sector funding (DH, 2002a; 2003a).

The Health Care Industries Task Force estimates that the total annual technology investment budget of the UK health industry at 2003/04 was £7.4 billion (2004). Of this, £5 billion was the estimated private sector investment (some £3.5 billion being attributable to pharmaceutical company research), £750 million was from charitable sources (approximately £500 million from the Wellcome Foundation) and £1.537 million was from public sector sources (£310 million for the Higher Education Finance Committee, mainly Medical Schools; £440 million for research councils, mainly the Medical Research Council; and £617 million for departmental research programmes, mainly the NHS). There are indications that very substantial investment – in both the science base of healthcare and in public health – has the potential to transform health in the first half of this century. The government notes that this investment will require public–private partnership, and a clear mechanism for directing and utilising such investment in order to improve the public health (DH, 2003b).

The subject of public–private partnership remains intensely contested. Pollock (2004) argues that it is not only uneconomic but undermines the basis of the NHS. The government's position is that the creation of a mixed economy of provision, with fair competition and transparent co-operation between public and private sectors, can bring greater creativity and advantages for both sides (HM Treasury, 2000). Maynard notes that the level and source of investment in further healthcare resources by public or private funding is less important than the direction of health and medical effort towards evidence-based practice in both public health and healthcare (Maynard, 2005).

While all three major political parties endorse the principle of public–private partnerships in England, the political climate for public–private partnership for investment is less welcoming in Scotland and Wales. This may prove a test of alternative policy futures with an increasingly mixed economy of healthcare provision in England and more reliance on public sector management in other home countries.

How the money should be spent

Over the long term, increased investment in healthcare has been associated with improved health outcomes in OECD countries (Or, 2000) and in WHO member states (Anand and Barnighausen, 2004). It is not true, however, that countries spending more on healthcare always achieve better health outcomes than those with lower levels of expenditure. Scotland, for example, spends some 18% more per capita and achieves worse health outcomes than England, and the US spends more than twice the level of England and still achieves worse health outcomes. Nolte and McKee (2004) recently carried out an exhaustive review, showing that in the 1990s only 16% of mortality in the UK was due to causes amenable to healthcare interventions. They suggest that beyond a certain level, the overall impact of further improvements in healthcare services or access on mortality is difficult to detect.

Thus, while it is necessary to invest in healthcare to meet public expectations, it is also important to develop public awareness that healthcare investment by itself cannot produce good health and that responsibility for managing health risks starts with the individual, the family and the community. This is not a message that can easily be delivered from government. It requires local leadership for health.

Within healthcare the National Institute for Clinical Excellence (NICE) has established a process for evaluating the evidence base, consulting with all parties and producing guidelines against which action by the NHS is assessed by the Health Commission. This is potentially a powerful lever to direct healthcare funding and improve clinical performance. The keys to its success over the next 15 years will be the capacity of NICE to complete guidance in all needed areas, the ability of the NHS and Healthcare Commission to ensure that guidance is followed by funding and implementation, and the perceived authority and competence of NICE and the health technology and economic assessment units with which it works.

NICE guidelines for economic evaluation as described by Sculpher (2004) are appropriate to clinical health technology assessment. However, these methods – which require the evaluation of the impact on Quality Adjusted Life Years (QALYs) measured in standard ways and modelling of the uncertainties of cause and effect – are much more difficult to apply to complex conditions such as multiple chronic diseases and mental illness. They are not relevant to long-term strategies for addressing the determinants of health. It will be difficult, but very important, to develop methodologies for Health Impact Assessment relevant to action on broader determinants of health.

A National Institute for Health and Clinical Excellence (NIHCE) is proposed in *Choosing Health* (DH, 2004d). It would be created by merging the National Institute for Clinical Excellence and the Health Development Agency. This body could play a very important role in advising on and directing funding for public health and addressing the wider determinants of health.

It is suggested that the new body should:

- produce a national plan for the health of the people along the lines of that developed by the National Institute of Public Health in Sweden (Ågren, 2003)
- advise on the shift in priorities and expenditure from acute treatment to long-term chronic conditions such as mental illness

- develop measures of community and individual health risk as a basis for investment for health and other decisions affecting health and environmental risks (for
  example nitrates, train protection and asbestos)
- advise on the use of measures of community health risk as a basis for funding PCT
  action on health protection and disease prevention
- advise on the costs and benefits of social marketing for health and different forms
  of local engagement and champions for health.

In all such matters it will be important for NIHCE to create a process to reach
consensus and a common understanding with representatives of the public and all
the agencies involved. The agency would benefit from a clear and independent
identity separate from the government but able to advise on health policy issues. It
will be important for this English agency to work closely with similar bodies in the
other home countries since there are aspects of health which require a UK-wide
approach.

At PCT or Health Board level, Directors of Public Health produce annual reports,
which are an important starting point for Health Improvement Plans and their
equivalent in other home countries (DH, 1998). These are intended to direct funding
and action by local authorities, health agencies and other local partners to improve
health. The reports and plans include measures of general and disease-specific
health status and risk, but at present there are few specific links to funding for action
on health determinants. In part this is because the evidence on the cost-effectiveness of
actions is often felt to be weak and of less pressing concern than other targets. It will
be important to address this funding issue, recognising that investments for health
are often longer term and more uncertain than investment in healthcare. It is
suggested that NIHCE (and its equivalent in other home countries) should monitor
investment for health and that impacts should be reviewed by the Healthcare
Commission.

The role of PCTs and GPs in commissioning services is crucial to the cost-
effectiveness of health spending in England. It seems likely that new agencies
will emerge to support specialist commissioning for people who require integrated
health and social care with significant elements of self-care. Integrated care commissioning may use new information and communication technology to monitor
and support patients and their carers. Such developments could learn from integrated care management in the US (Lawrence, 2002).

Policy recommendations

Over the next 15 years, it will be essential to ensure that the government is able to
address the full costs to society of health and to engage with all sectors. A new
Health of the People Act should express the responsibilities of all parties for health
and their rights to health and healthcare (Monaghan *et al.*, 2003).

Departments of Health in other home countries have the advantages of smaller
scale and a common structure of local authorities and health agencies. They are
pursuing different development paths, which create opportunities to learn from
experience. This is particularly relevant to the success or failure of public–private
partnerships.

Detailed proposals for the future funding of health include the following:

- the NHS will be funded primarily through taxation, but must develop resilience to manage resources in an era of cost containment
- other sources of funding including co-payment, private insurance, product taxes and employer contributions to occupational health should be examined and evidence of their effectiveness and impact on health equity reviewed
- long-term residential care should be funded from a system of public insurance supplemented by private insurance linked to pensions, property ownership and inheritance
- Primary Care Trusts should be developed as community-owned health maintenance organisations with incentives for investment for health
- measures should be taken to support and strengthen the commissioning function, including innovations in commissioning integrated care
- local authority and health agency boundaries should be aligned, and must work together to address long-term physical, mental and social care needs
- taxes and subsidies should be used to support healthy choices by making healthy foods and activities cheaper in relation to non-healthy choices
- The National Institute for Health and Clinical Excellence (NIHCE) should advise on cross-sector policy and funding and produce a national plan for health
- NIHCE should also advise on investment in social marketing for health and develop clear links with, and ownership by, local champions for health
- information services should be strengthened to educate, inform and empower people to make healthy choices for spending and consumption
- industry-based programmes for occupational health should be developed by championing best practice and possibly some form of regulation and levy
- Dutch and German experience of patient-held budgets should be examined and introduced to support long-term care, including support for informal care
- new initiatives should be supported to improve integrated care provision and commissioning for people with complex physical/mental/social care needs
- a unified process to identify, research and take action on unhealthy products and practices, should be introduced, funded by producers and retailers
- health status improvement should be measured and used at a community level as a basis for investment for health and to support personal health choices
- national accounts for health should be extended to recognise the full cost of health to society and health as a global public good.

In reflecting on these proposals it may be helpful to pose the question, 'Who is going to pay the price of lack of investment in health?' In the US, experts are predicting that the current generation of school children will live shorter and unhealthier lives than their parents, as a result of obesity, poor diet, lifestyle and inequality (Brownell, 2004; Jacobs and Morone, 2004). In the UK, a similar case has been made (Stoate, 2004). While it seems more likely that average life expectancy will continue to rise in the UK, increasing rates of obesity and lack of engagement with health amongst lower social-economic groups will mean that the poor will continue to bear the greatest burden of ill health unless public health measures are greatly improved.

References

Ableson P (2003) *Returns on Investment in Public Health.* Department of Health and Ageing, Government of Australia, Canberra.

Acheson D (1998) *Report of the Independent Inquiry into Inequalities in Health.* The Stationery Office, London.

Ågren G (2003) *Sweden's New Public Health Policy.* Swedish National Institute for Public Health, Sandviken.

Alcohol Concern (2000) Alcohol problems costing Britain £3.3 billion. http://www.alcohol concern.org.uk/servlets/doc/282. Accessed: 4 October 2004.

Anand S and Barnighausen T (2004) Human resources and health outcomes: cross-country econometric study. *The Lancet.* **364**(9445): 1558–60.

ASH (2004) Factsheet no.16: the economics of tobacco. http://www.ash.org.uk/html/factsheets/html/fact16.html. Accessed: 4 October 2004.

BBC (2004) Free personal care 'costing more'. http://news.bbc.co.uk/1/hi/scotland/3696738.stm. Accessed: 28 September 2004.

Beatty C and Fothergill S (2004) *The Diversion from Unemployment to Sickness across British Regions and Districts.* Centre for Economic and Social Research, Sheffield Hallam University, Sheffield.

Bell B and Smith J (2004) *Health Disability Insurance and Labour Force Participation. Working paper 218.* Bank of England, London.

Bell G (2003) *A presentation by Gavin Bell, President of the Proprietary Association of Great Britain.* Proprietary Association of Great Britain, London.

Bosanquet N, Browne A, Bull A, Day G, Desai M, Disney H, Green DG, Irvine B, Lea R, Lees C, Neil A, Ormerod P, Pollard S, Smith S and Young M (2003)*The Final Report of the Health Policy Consensus Group: a new consensus for NHS reform.* Civitas, London.

Brown G (2002) *Speech on Economic Stability and Strong Public Services: the Social Market Foundation.* HM Treasury, London.

Brownell K (2004) *Food Fight.* Yale Center for Eating and Weight Disorders and McGraw Hill, New York.

Brundtland GH (2000) *Health and Population: Reith Lecture 4, Respect for the Earth series.* BBC, London.

Burke S, Gray I, Paterson K and JM (2002) *Environmental Health 2012: a key partner in delivering the public health agenda.* Health Development Agency, London.

Butterworth S (2003) *Making the Connection: trading standards contribution to public health.* Trading Standards Institute, London.

Carers UK (2002) *Without Us ...? Calculating the value of carers' support.* Carers UK, London.

CBI (2004) *CBI Press Release.* Central Business Institute, London.

Chancellor of the Exchequer (2002) Chancellor of the Exchequer's Budget statement – 17 April 2002. http://www.hm-treasury.gov.uk/budget/bud_bud02/bud_bud02_speech.cfm. Accessed: 3 October 2004.

Citizens Advice Bureau (2001) *Unhealthy Charges: charging for health.* Citizens Advice Bureau, London.

Cottam H and Leadbeater C (2004) *Red Paper 01 Health: co-creating Services.* Design Council, London.

Coulter A and Magee H (2003) *The European Patient of the Future.* Open University Press, McGraw Hill, Berkshire.

CREDES (2002) *OECD Health Database.* CREDES, Paris.

Dargie C (2000) *Policy Futures for UK Health. 2000 Report.* The Nuffield Trust, London.

DCMS (2004) *Prime Minister Announces Massive Boost for School Sports.* Press release. Department for Culture, Media and Sport, London.

DEFRA (2003) *Implementing the Nitrates Directive: how should England implement the 1991 nitrates directive: a consultation*. Department for Environment Food and Rural Affairs, London.

DH (1996) *Patient's Charter: monitoring guide rights and other standards – a consolidated guide*. Department of Health, London.

DH (1998) *Local Plans to Improve Health Throughout England*. Department of Health, London.

DH (2000a) *The NHS Plan: a plan for investment, a plan for reform. Cmnd 4818-I*. Department of Health, London.

DH (2000b) *The NHS Plan: the Government's response to the royal commission on long-term care 2000*. The Stationery Office, London.

DH (2001) *National School Fruit Scheme Evaluation*. Department of Health, London.

DH (2002a) *Department of Health Investment Programme 2002–03*. Department of Health, London.

DH (2002b) *Delivering the NHS Plan: next steps on investment, next steps on reform*. Department of Health, London.

DH (2003a) *A Vision for Pharmacy in the NHS*. The Stationery Office, London.

DH (2003b) *Our Inheritance, Our Future: realising the potential of genetics in the NHS. Cmnd 5791-II*. Department of Health, London.

DH (2004a) *Chief Executive's Report to the NHS December 2004*. Department of Health, London.

DH (2004b) *Payment by Results Preparing for 2005: consultation outcome*. Department of Health, London.

DH (2004c) *New Health Programme Trial to Improve Older Patient Care*. Press release. Department of Health, London.

DH (2004d) *Choosing Health: making healthier choices easier. Cmnd 6374*. Department of Health, London.

DH (2004e) *Making Partnerships Work for Patients' Carers and Service Users. Gateway ref. 3703*. Department of Health, London.

DH (2004f) *Choose and Book: patient choice of hospital and booked appointment*. Department of Health, London.

DH (2004g) *Health Information on Your TV Screen*. Press release. Department of Health, London.

DH (2004h) *Growing Capacity Independent Sector Diagnostic and Treatment Centres: list of national and local procurement scheme details*. The Stationery Office, London.

DH (2004i) *List of NHS LIFT Schemes*. The Stationery Office, London.

Donaldson C and Gerard K (1989) Countering moral hazard in public and private healthcare systems: a review of recent evidence. *Journal of Social Policy*. **18**(2): 235–51.

DWP (2005) *Pathways to Work: helping people into employment: consultative paper*. Department of Work and Pensions, London.

Evans R (2002) Financing healthcare taxation and the alternatives. In: E Mossialos, A Dixon, J Figueras and J Kutzin (eds) *Funding Health Care: options for Europe*. Oxford University Press, Oxford.

Evans R (2005) Political wolves and economic sheep; the sustainability of public health insurance in Canada. In: A Maynard (ed.) *The Public–Private Mix for Health*. Radcliffe Publishing, Oxford.

FCO (1999) *Britain's Sports and Fitness Industry*. Foreign and Commonwealth Office, London.

Gooday I (2000) *A Survey of the Control of Asbestos at Work Regulations*. Health and Safety Commission, London.

Gray DP (1995) *Primary care and the public health. Harben Lecture: Health and Hygiene*. The Royal Institute of Public Health and Hygiene, London.

Hamilton W, Round A and Sharp D (1999) Effect on hospital attendance rates of giving patients a copy of their referral letter: a randomised controlled trial. *British Medical Journal*. **318**: 1395.

Harrison S and Moran M (2000) Resources and rationing: managing supply and demand in health care. In: G Albrecht, R Fitzpatrick and S Scrimshaw (eds) *Handbook of Social Studies in Health and Medicine*. Sage, London, pp. 493–503.

Hasler P and Cooney A (2002) *Understanding the Health and Fitness Market*. MORI, London.

HDA (2003) *Drug Use Prevention: a review of reviews*. Health Development Agency, London.

Health and Safety Commission (1999) *Report on Improving Access to Occupational Health Support*. Health and Safety Commission, London.

Healthcare Industries Task Force (2004) *HITF Working Group 2: R&D and the Industrial Base Little Working Group – a few 'big hits'*. Healthcare Industries Task Force, London.

HM Treasury (2000) *Public–Private Partnerships: the Government's approach*. The Stationery Office, London.

HM Treasury (2001) *Long-term Care Insurance: consultation*. The Stationery Office, London.

House of Commons Health Committee (2004) *Obesity. Third Report of Session 2003–04*. House of Commons Health Committee, London.

Jacobs LR and Morone J (2004) *Health and wealth*. http://www.prospect.org/web/page.ww?section=root&name=ViewPrint&articleId=7755. Accessed: 3 October 2004.

Johnson M (2004) *The expert patient programme: Speech to the Expert Patients Programme and Long-term Medical Conditions Alliance*. TSO, London.

Kickbusch I and Payne L (2003) Twenty-first century health promotion: the public health revolution meets the wellness revolution. *Health Promotion International*. 18(4): 275–8.

Kickbusch I and Payne L (2004) *Constructing Global Health in the 21st Century: global governance and accountability*. Harvard University, Cambridge, MA.

Lawrence D (2002) *From Chaos to Care: the promise of team-based medicine*. Perseus Books, Cambridge.

LGA, The UK Public Health Association and The NHS Confederation (2004) *Realising the Potential for the Public's Health*. The Local Government Association, London.

Lister G (2005) Health policy futures and cost scenarios for England 2003–2023. In: S Dawson and C Sausman (eds) *Future Health Organisations and Systems*. Palgrave Macmillan, Basingstoke.

Lister G, Ingram A and Prowle M (2005) Case study: UK financing of international cooperation for health. In: I Kaul and P Conceição (eds) *The New Public Finance: responding to global challenges*. Oxford University Press, New York.

Machin D and McShane D (2001) *Providing Free Personal Care for Older People: research commissioned to inform the work of the care development group*. The Scottish Executive Central Research Unit, Edinburgh.

Maynard A (2005) *The Public–Private Mix for Health*. Radcliffe Publishing, Oxford.

Mintel International Group Ltd (2003) *Reduced Fat and Reduced Calorie Food UK*. Mintel International Group Ltd, London.

Monaghan S, Huws D and Navarro M (2003) *The Case for a New UK Health of the People Act*. The Nuffield Trust, London.

Mossialos E, Dixon A, Figueras J and Kutzin J (2002) *Policy Brief No. 4: Funding Health Care: options for Europe*. The European Observatory on Health Care Systems, Copenhagen.

Mossialos E and Le Grand J (1999) *Health Care and Cost Containment in the EU*. Ashgate, Aldershot.

Mossialos E and Thomson S (2004) *Voluntary Health Insurance in the European Union*. European Observatory on Health Care Systems and Policies, Brussels.

Nolte E and McKee M (2004) *Does Healthcare Save Lives*. The Nuffield Trust, London.

Office of the Deputy Prime Minister (2003) *Local Government Act 2003*. The Stationery Office, London.

ONS (2002) *Health and Safety Statistics Highlights 2001/2*. Office of National Statistics, London. Accessed: 4 October 2004. www.statistics.gov.uk.

ONS (2004a) *Environmental Accounts: spring 2004 edition*. Office of National Statistics, London. www.statistics.gov.uk. Accessed: 3 October 2004.

ONS (2004b) *Health Expectancy: living longer, more years in poor health*. Office of National Statistics, London.

ONS (2004c) *UK Health Accounts*. Office of National Statistics, London.

Or Z (2000) *Exploring the Effects of Health Care on Mortality Across OECD Countries*. OECD, Paris.

PACTS (2000) *Road Safety Spending in Great Britain: who stands to gain? Research brief RB/100*. Parliamentary Advisory Council for Transport Safety, London.

Perlman F and Gray S (2004) *The Specialist Public Health Workforce in the UK: a report for the Board of the Faculty of Public Health*. Faculty of Public Health, London.

Phillips WM, Bridgemen J and Ferguson-Smith M (2000) *The BSE Inquiry*. The Stationery Office, London.

Pilzer PZ (2002) *The Wellness Revolution: how to make a fortune in the next trillion dollar industry*. John Wiley and Sons, New York.

Pollock AM (2004) *NHS Plc: the privatisation of our health care*. Verso, London.

Proprietary Association of Great Britain (2003) *Annual Report*. Proprietary Association of Great Britain, London.

Reinhardt UE (2001) Commentary: on the apocalypse of the retiring baby boom. *Canadian Journal of Aging*. **20**(1): 192–204.

Robinson R (2002) User charges for health care. In: E Mossialos, A Dixon, J Figueras and J Kutzin (eds) *Funding Health Care: options for Europe*. Oxford University Press, Oxford.

Robson S (2004) *Chairman's Report of the Occupational Health Committee 2004*. British Medical Association, London.

Saltman RB and Figueras JF (1998) Analyzing the evidence on European health reforms. *Health Affairs*. **17**(2): 85–108.

Sculpher M (2004) *Economic Evaluation for NICE. 5th European Conference on Health Economics*. London School of Economics, London.

Social Market Foundation (2003) *Private Payment for Health Boon or Bane: the Social Market Foundation Report*. Social Market Foundation, London.

Staricoff RL (2004) *Arts in Health: a review of the medical literature. Research Report 36*. Arts Council, London.

Stoate H (2004) *All's Well that Starts Well*. Fabian Society, London.

Sutherland S (1999) *With Respect to Old Age: long-term care rights and responsibilities*. The Stationery Office, London.

Tuohy CH, Flood CM and Stabile M (2004) How does private finance affect public health care systems? Marshalling the evidence from OECD nations. *Journal of Health Politics, Policy and Law*. **29**(3): 359–96.

Turning Point (2004) Turning 40. http://www.turning-point.co.uk/NR/rdonlyres/64B6F401-3C9D-4853-AB88-5E6733090FCC/0/Turning40.pdf. Accessed: 4 October 2004.

Uff J and Cullen WD (2001) *The Joint Inquiry into Train Protection Systems*. Health and Safety Commission, London.

Wanless D (2002) *Securing our Future Health: taking a long-term view*. HM Treasury, London.

Wanless D (2003) *Securing Good Health for the Whole Population – population health trends*. HM Treasury, London.

Wanless D (2004) *Securing Good Health for the Whole Population. Final Report*. HM Treasury, London.

WHO (1946) *Preamble to the Constitution of the World Health Organization*. Adopted by the International Health Conference, New York, 19–22 June.

Wiener JM, Hixon Illston L and Hanley RJ (1994) *Sharing the Burden: strategies for public and private long-term care insurance*. Brookings Institute, Washington.

Wittenberg R, Comas-Herrera A, Pickard L and Hancock R (2002a) *Future Demand for Long-term Care in the UK: a summary of projections of long-term care finance for older people to 2051*. Joseph Rowntree Foundation, York.

Wittenberg R, Sandhu B and Knapp M (2002b) Funding long-term care: the public and private options. In: E Mossialos, A Dixon, J Figueras and J Kutzin (eds) *Funding Health Care: options for Europe*. Oxford University Press, Oxford.

Woodhouse K (2000) *Report of the Wales Care Strategy Group 2000*. Assembly for Wales, Cardiff.

Part 3

Conclusions

Chapter 9

Where are the linkages for joined-up policy?

Sandra Dawson in association with Raj Bhopal, Graham Lister, Zoë Slote Morris, Suzanne Wait and Ron Zimmern

As the *Policy Futures for UK Health* project progressed, the danger of looking at key policy areas as discrete themes became evident. Part of the consultation process involved asking participants to identify cross-cutting themes. Five policy areas were identified as germane to all the chapters. They are:

- the determinants of health
- equity and equality
- individual and community expectations of healthcare and health
- science, technology and industrial policy
- information, evaluation and benchmarking.

This chapter outlines these themes and provides some illustrative examples.

Determinants of health

Among the factors influencing health and disease in a population are environment, lifestyle, hereditary and intrinsic factors, as well as healthcare services (Blum, 1981; Evans and Stoddart, 1990; 1994; Labonte, 1993; Lalonde, 1974; Mausner and Kramer, 1985). These are discussed in greater detail below.

Environmental factors

Environmental factors can be organised into two categories: pre-natal and post-natal. Pre-natal factors predict adult health. Maternal illness, smoking, alcoholism, high blood pressure, poor socio-economic conditions and multiple pregnancies all predict low birth weight and thus adult poor health. Relevant factors in the post-natal environment include the 'physical, chemical and biological environment', as well as the 'social, psychological and economic environment' (Monaghan *et al.*, 2003). Physical, chemical and biological risks are strongly associated with social class, largely through occupation (Barker *et al.*, 1991). Environmental risk factors include access to nutritious food, pure water and the effective disposal of sewage, environmental pollution and housing. Dampness, lack of heating and wall-to-wall carpeting have been associated with respiratory disorders (Best, 1995), while over-crowding and the broader social environment are also relevant (Last, 1998; Macintyre *et al.*, 1993; Patrick and Wickizer, 1995).

Social, psychological and economic environmental factors include the central issue of socio-economic inequality, which some consider to be the most important determinant of health inequalities (Davey-Smith *et al.*, 1997; Townsend *et al.*, 1992; Whitehead, 1995). Besides material differences by socio-economic group, relative inequality and social exclusion (Marmot *et al.*, 1995; Wilkinson, 1997; Wilkinson, 1996), worse health outcomes are related to stress, lack of social support (Berkman and Syme, 1979) and community cohesion (Halpern, 1995; Patrick and Wickizer, 1995). Lower socio-economic status is also associated with greater exposure to environmental risks, in turn associated with ill health. Those with lower socio-economic status are more likely to experience unemployment and dangerous occupations. They more often have low control over their work (Hallqvist *et al.*, 1998) and poor education. Lower socio-economic status is also associated with riskier 'lifestyle choices' (Brenner, 1995; Davey-Smith *et al.*, 1997).

Lifestyle factors

Lifestyle factors are well rehearsed in contemporary policy and media. Cade *et al.* (1988) suggest that diet in adulthood may be less important than diet in childhood. Fruit and vegetables are believed to have a protective effect against bowel disease and cancer while fatty acids and salt cause heart disease and stroke (James *et al.*, 1997). A related issue is lack of exercise and obesity, which predict coronary heart disease. Smoking, alcohol and drug misuse predict health status (Bunker, 2001).

Hereditary and intrinsic factors

In terms of hereditary and intrinsic factors, the most important factor is age, though gender is also relevant. The importance of genetics to many areas of health is still not clear although genes are implicated in a range of diseases. For some of these, such as breast cancer, treatment can be attempted by conventional medical methods while for others, such as Huntington's disease and cystic fibrosis, there is no currently available treatment (Lenaghan, 1998; Zimmern and Cook, 2000). Alzheimer's disease, some heart disease and diabetes are also thought to include genetic elements (Lenaghan, 1998).

Healthcare services

There is debate about the contribution of healthcare services to health (McKeown, 1979). Hobbs and Jamrozik (2004) suggest that social, environmental and public health interventions are more effective ways of securing health gain than medical services. Bunker (2001) suggests that half of the increase in life expectancy can be attributed to medical care. There have been improvements within medicine – Monaghan *et al.* (2003) cite childhood leukaemia and testicular cancer as examples – but as these diseases are rare, the population effect appears small.

Since determinants are linked, policy responses need to be sufficiently sophisticated. Two challenges discussed below highlight the ever-present theme of the changing relationship of the individual and the state, but also draw on issues relevant to disease, care and the costs of health.

The determinants of health in joined-up policy

The state expects individuals to 'self-care', to make healthy lifestyle choices and therefore to possess the means to act 'responsibly'. This expectation naturally implies a measure of individual agency and autonomy (Secretary of State for Health, 1999). The problem with this is that it fails to locate individuals as embedded in a socio-economic reality partly determined by state policy: individuals are not entirely autonomous and free to change behaviour and choose healthier lifestyles (Vallgarda, 2001).

Fixed circumstances often limit choice since poorer or more deprived individuals may not have the opportunity or encouragement from their environments to change their behaviours. Poorer neighbourhoods, for example, are likely to have more alcohol outlets, while healthy foods are likely to be more expensive or unavailable (Vallgarda, 2001). There are also fewer exercise facilities in poorer areas. Unhealthy lifestyle behaviours may be interpreted as a means of coping with deprivation (Brocklehurst and Costello, 2003; Vlad, 2003) because they often represent the easiest and most affordable choices. For this reason, unhealthy consumption patterns are likely to persist among the poor (Moore, 1999). Wilkinson remarks, 'Because behaviour is socially determined, individuals can only be changed by a changing society' (1996).

Reducing incidence and mortality of disease through action on health determinants within society would fundamentally impact on overall disease rates. It would have the potential to reduce levels of chronic illness and morbidity. The question that follows is whether lifestyle choices trigger forms of healthcare rationing.

Reducing health inequalities on a broader societal scale would be optimal (Klein, 2003), but it is uncertain whether the government is willing to spend (Brocklehurst and Costello, 2003) and, by implication, raise sufficient funds. There is presently concern that money is not being invested into public health research unless a crisis demands it (Frank *et al.*, 2003; Wellcome Trust, 2004), such as in the case of infectious diseases. Evaluations of public health interventions are rare (Dargie, 2000; DH, 2004; Wanless, 2004). The Medical Research Council, for example, allocates less than 4% to public health research (Millward *et al.*, 2003).

Equity and equality

Health inequalities can be defined as differences in health status or in the distribution of health determinants between different population groups – differences in mobility between elderly people and younger populations, for example, or differences in mortality rates between people from different social classes (Barnes, 2004). Some health inequalities are attributable to biological variations or individual choice, others to the external environment and conditions mainly outside the control of the individuals concerned. In the UK, for instance, the South Asian population is typically less prone to cancer, but more prone to heart disease and diabetes when compared with other ethnic groups (Cappuccio *et al.*, 2002; Gill *et al.*, in press).

Health inequities, on the other hand, have a moral or ethical dimension relating to fairness and justice: 'inequity refers to differences in health which are not only unnecessary and avoidable, but in addition are considered unfair and unjust'

(Whitehead, 1992). Equity in health therefore implies that everyone should have a fair opportunity to attain their full health potential and, more pragmatically, that no one should be disadvantaged from achieving this potential if it can be avoided (Barnes, 2004). In practice, equity is usually associated with creating equal opportunities for health and with bringing health inequalities down to the lowest possible level (Barnes, 2004; Hamer *et al.*, 2003).

There is naturally a close relationship between the two concepts. If, for example, inequalities in health (namely, an uneven distribution in health outcome) are unnecessary and avoidable, then they may also be considered unjust and unfair. If the relatively high prevalence of diabetes in the South Asian UK population results from biological factors or individual choices related to diet and lifestyle, for example, this can be considered a health inequality. If, however, this unusually high rate of disease can be attributed to poorer access to healthcare or inferior disease management, this must also be considered a health inequity (Britton *et al.*, 2004). Not all health inequalities are also inequities. Older people are, on average, unavoidably less healthy than the young (a health inequality), but because this is impossible to change, we cannot consider it an inequity. A denial of services based on age, however, could be inequitable.

Nevertheless, the issue of the definition is complicated because the precise meaning and importance of equity will depend on subjective factors such as cultural beliefs and attitudes (City University London, 2004). These include:

- how inequalities are explained
- the values underpinning the healthcare system (libertarian versus egalitarian)
- whether focus is placed on horizontal (preferential treatment for those with greater health needs) or vertical equity (equal treatment for equivalent needs)
- how finance is arranged (whether a funding system is regressive, progressive or proportional)
- how equitable distribution of care is.

Concepts of equity relevant to the distribution of care include:

- utilitarianism
- equality of health outcomes
- equality of expenditure
- equality of use for equal need
- equality of access for equal need.

As a consequence, an understanding of the values and objectives of the healthcare system must be achieved prior to assessments of equity.

Implications for these debates are examined here in relation to the themes of governance and the evaluation of performance, and self-care.

Equity and equality in joined-up policy

Governments continually have to deal with competing demands for public funds, and this necessitates careful use of scarce resources. Before they take action, they must consider which means are most appropriate for reducing health inequities and how best to measure successful intervention. Should success to be measured in absolute terms, by judging the reduction in the gap between the best- and worst-off in society, or in relative terms, by judging the degree to which the worst-off have improved relative to where they started? In view of the difficulty in leveling health status across populations, should governments accept that not only is health inequality unavoidable, but that a certain level of health inequity will always persist? Should inequity refer to access or outcome?

Whether self-care increases health inequality and inequity remains to be seen. Since self-care is based on access to information and care networks in addition to self-efficacy, it may lead to the most disadvantaged becoming more disadvantaged. For better-informed and expert patients, access to information could make the relationship between patients and medical staff more equitable. If the balance swings strongly to self-care individual, market power will become more important. People's willingness and eagerness for private care will impact on equity and access.

Individual and community expectations of healthcare and health

Since the UK spends below the trend line for EU countries, it is to be expected that the UK public will be relatively dissatisfied with healthcare (Lister, 2005) – and they are (Mossialos, 1997). In 1982, Maxwell showed that the proportion of GDP that countries choose to spend on healthcare can be predicted from the level of GDP per capita (Maxwell, 1982). The question is whether increasing expenditure in the UK to match the levels of EU countries of similar wealth, as proposed over the next five years, will result in greater satisfaction. Research suggests that there is no direct correlation between the level of expenditure and overall healthcare performance (Appleby and Rosete, 2003; Social Services and Public Safety for NI, 2001).

Social trends data indicate that the proportion of people satisfied with hospital services remained steady between 1996 and 1998, rose in 1999 and 2000, and then fell in 2001 and 2002 – to only just over 50% of people saying they were satisfied with hospital services (ONS, 2004). Satisfaction levels were much higher for those who had recently been hospital patients and for older people (who are more likely to have been patients). Satisfaction with GP services is consistently higher than for hospitals, with higher levels of satisfaction amongst those who had recently visited their doctor.

Public expectation of healthcare is not simply for better services. Commentators suggest that patients are increasingly behaving as consumers, demanding greater levels of autonomy and choice (Coulter, 2002; Coulter and Magee, 2003; Dargie, 2000). It is not clear what relative value is placed on the availability of a local government-owned hospital – as compared to services received from a distant privately-owned or even foreign hospital. Studies show, however, that satisfaction with such treatments are comparable to those of local hospital users (Lowson *et al.*, 2002). This suggests that people care less about the provider than the service they receive.

Central forecasts of the demand for long-term care have assumed increasing unit costs but do not include provision for increasing expectations of standards and choice with rising GDP per capita (Wittenberg *et al.*, 2002). It is also apparent that a major source of dissatisfaction with current long-term care services is their frag-mented and inflexible nature (Turning Point, 2004). Much emphasis has been placed on the delay or compression of the period of ill-health (Association of

Directors of Social Services, 2000) but Kirkwood suggests the scope for compression is limited (2001). This may lead to increasing dissatisfaction with the quality, nature and outcome of long-term care.

One approach to resolving this, adopted in The Netherlands, has been to give budgets to patients and let them choose their service package and care providers (Dekkers and Lister, 2002). Similar proposals are made in the current Green Paper, *Independence, Well-being and Choice: our vision for the future of social care for adults in England* (DH, 2005). The Joseph Rowntree Foundation recently published a review of long-term care funding in the UK, drawing on international experience, stating that there is a limit to funding long-term care since there are other economic pressures (Glendinning *et al.*, 2004).

Expectations for personal health may also rise with increasing wealth. They continue to divide across the inequity gap, with the poorest expecting, and getting, worse health and healthcare services. At the same time, those who are better-off demand higher levels of support for personal health maintenance, with more choice and better standards of service in healthcare (Opinion Leader Research, 2004).

Until recently, England was the only country in Europe with no real democratic involvement in health below national government. This may be one cause of a decline in social capital and trust in government (Rothstein, 2004). Local democratic involvement in health decisions can express majority values but health is also a right of those who have minority interests, both by the nature of their health needs and by reason of ethnicity or other cause. Public and patient involvement must express both majority and minority needs and expectations (CPPIH, 2004; Farrell, 2004).

While policy in a democracy cannot operate purely on the basis of public expectation, at the same time it cannot be ignored. This leads to the question of how health expectations can and should be measured. Existing measures, including patient satisfaction, are not necessarily suitable to assess the 'user perspective' (Holland *et al.*, 1998; Mossialos, 1997). A future challenge is to develop more sensitive and contextual measures.

Individual and community expectations of healthcare and health in joined-up policy

Different perceptions of health and self-assessments of health status may be related in part to different expectations for health (Salomon *et al.*, 2004). The perception of health could also be described as the gap between expectations and experience of health (Carr *et al.*, 2001). People with the same clinical condition, but with different expectations, will report a different quality of life. Some people, because of their experiences, have low expectations of health. Carr *et al.* (2001) suggest that the core objective of health promotion is to change people's expectations, but they also point out that by changing people's expectations of health, their perception of quality of life could ostensibly decrease. As patients become more informed and aware about healthcare choices, their growing awareness will lead to higher expectations. The important question is whether rising expectations or better information will lead to better health outcomes.

A combination of rising expectations and increasing reliance on self-care is likely to mean an expansion in health choices. A particular contemporary issue is the increasing array and popularity of complementary and alternative therapy available. The drive for complementary and alternative medicine (CAM) has often resulted either from a situation in which patients are not satisfied with conventional healthcare concerning the treatment and the experience of care, or because CAM is more in line with their own values and beliefs regarding health (Astin, 1998).

Science, technology and industrial policy

The ability to prevent and treat illness requires both an understanding of disease processes and the availability of technologies, such as diagnostic tests and pharmaceutical agents. The way in which science is conducted and the factors contributing to innovation are crucial elements among the many structural mechanisms and policy considerations that determine the health of the population. Mechanisms that lie outside the health system can have significant influences upon it. These may include the processes by which research is funded, the laws that regulate technology transfer and intellectual property, the fiscal regimes imposed on the commercial sector and the principles that underpin notions of consent and confidentiality in research practice.

These matters have been the subject of discussion and debate within the scientific and medical communities, and across the biotechnology and pharmaceutical industries, for many years. The Pharmaceutical Industry Competitiveness Task Force (PICTF), which published its final report in March 2001, was perhaps the start of a more formal process for their consideration. Since then, a plethora of policy documents and statements have been issued, including:

- *Science and Innovation – working towards a ten-year investment framework* (DTI, Treasury and DfES, March 2004)
- *White Paper: our inheritance, our future – realising the potential of genetics in the NHS* (DH, June 2003)
- *Research for Patient Benefit Working Party* (DH, March 2004)
- *Bioscience 2015: improving national wealth, improving national health* (Bioscience IGT and BIA, supported by DTI, DH, November 2003)
- *Lambert Review of Business–University Collaboration* (HM Treasury, December 2003)
- *Strengthening Clinical Research* (Academy of Medical Sciences, October 2003)
- *Securing Good Health for the Whole Population* (HM Treasury and DH, February 2004)
- *Public Health Sciences: challenges and opportunities* (Wellcome Trust, March 2004).

Together these texts emphasise some common points:

- the importance of genetics and molecular science research
- the need for a vibrant research base and research capacity within the UK
- the imperative of having strong and well-developed links and collaborations between academia, the NHS and the commercial sector

- the importance of the NHS as a unique resource for clinical trials and all forms of clinical research including epidemiological studies and health service research
- the growing importance of public health and preventive medicine
- the necessity of having an appropriate and balanced regulatory regime for the conduct of research.

Biomedical sciences have the potential to impact on health over the coming decades. The legislative, regulatory and policy regimes discussed in the documents above will have an impact on how scientific advances and technology develop and how these in turn lead to interventions that benefit human health and increase the wealth of the nation. Simultaneously, they raise a series of issues that need to be addressed.

Science, technology and industrial policy in joined-up policy

Policy in this area is premised on an explicit need to be joined-up. The focus should be on funding and regulation, as well as the responsibility of different agencies regarding performance measures and incentives. Once pure science enters into a phase of applied research and clinical development, it needs a greater inter-disciplinary focus. The Research Assessment Exercise (RAE) of UK Higher Education Institutions, however, is structured in ways that do not necessarily support this imperative.

The allocation of research funding raises another dilemma. Is the system to encourage 'excellence or equity'? Should research monies go to places that are 'excellent' and will deliver higher returns for the money, or should they be distributed by some other 'social' and political criteria across the country? The view of the Science Technology and Industrial Policy workshop at the Policy Futures for UK Health Consultation Conference was that investment for excellence should prevail, although it should be tempered to ensure at least some degree of uniform provision.

Another aspect of research funding that requires consideration is the funding gap between early basic research (publicly-funded) and major product development (industry-funded). Between the two, as research enters a developmental phase, funding is required to establish 'proof of principle'. It is often difficult, if not impossible, to secure funding for this purpose. Policy needs to address how this gap is filled, and how the public and private sectors might work in partnership to this end.

The state is aware of the need to provide a legislative and policy framework that allows for innovation, while taking into account the values and preferences of the society in which the scientific process is embedded. This can be seen in recent legislation on the use of human tissue or of guidance and regulation in the use of stem cells. Also relevant here are issues of intellectual property rights and the extent to which the current system of patent protection provides the right balance between encouraging commercial developments and securing benefits for the public's health.

The state has a responsibility to regulate commercial interests in a manner that will reassure the public, which is currently untrusting of industry and averse to certain aspects of technological development (Stratford et al., 1999; The Royal Society and Royal Academy of Engineering, 2003). The state needs to provide evidence that public money spent on development is being put to best effect, and that it is spent on social as much as economic outcomes. The tension between commercial objectives and public health values is real and needs to be explicitly managed. It is no longer appropriate to hold the view that this relationship is one of bad versus good. Ways must be found to bring the two together.

Concerns regarding the relationship between commercial organisations and clinicians need to be addressed since government policy demands a much closer relationship between the commercial sector and both academia and the NHS. Should commercial organisations be encouraged to develop products that will then not be bought by the UK? Are there innovative ways in which government, the NHS and entrepreneurs can work together to reduce the effect of these tensions on the economy? Or ways in which products can be developed to address the actual burden of disease and allow more people to stay at home?

Information, evaluation and benchmarking

A driving force behind all health policy is a desire to improve health status and to manage healthcare costs effectively, with demonstrable improvements in quality of care and quality of life. The bedrock of any policy development must be measurement and evaluation. In recent times, greater emphasis has been placed on integrating the collection and evaluation of data at national, regional and local level. Results thus far have been patchy and this is an area for substantial and sustained development in the future. The publications of Leatherman and Sutherland (2003, 2005) are major landmarks in documenting performance in UK health.

Following the scandals of Harold Shipman and the Bristol Royal Infirmary, in order to improve accountability and quality, the government invested significantly in boosting health information systems. It encouraged systematic evaluation of health outcomes and benchmarking of health system performance (Blalock, 1999; DH, 1997a). England launched 'the most ambitious, comprehensive and intentionally funded national initiative to improve healthcare quality in the world' (Leatherman and Sutherland, 2003). Similar trends occurred in Wales, Scotland and Northern Ireland (DH and Social Services and Public Safety for Northern Ireland, 2002; Economic Policy Unit, 2003; Health Information in Wales, 2003; Perfomance Assessment Network, 2004). Five years after the publication of the NHS Plan (DH, 2000), it seems reasonable to ask whether the focus on information, evaluation and benchmarking has paid off.[1]

In January this year, the Shipman Inquiry (Smith J, 2005) concluded that '[before 2000] local PCOs [Primary Care Organisations] did not have monitoring systems in place that might have enabled them to detect the aberrant conduct of a doctor such as Shipman'. This begs the question of whether the reforms in place today will safeguard the quality of care in the future. More broadly, is the information

---

[1] Health information may be seen to include: all data on disease, treatment options and health risks and outcomes; public health and the functioning of the healthcare system in general. For the purposes of this chapter, 'information' is considered within the narrow confines of indicator data on processes, quality, outcomes and performance that are produced for the purposes of government-driven benchmarking efforts. Similarly, whilst recognising that not all evaluative data are used for benchmarking purposes, our discussion addresses mainly information used for national benchmarking purposes in an effort to focus discussions. For a broader discussion of these topics, see Wait (2004), Nolte *et al.* (2005) and Wait and Nolte (in press).

being collected useful for evaluation purposes? Are evaluation and benchmarking guiding policy? What can be done to strengthen this process? What are the implications for future policy recommendations? This chapter addresses each of these questions.

What do we know about the quality of care at present?

One of the main reasons for recent benchmarking initiatives has been to improve the quality of care (DH, 1997b). The first Wanless report (2002) suggested that the UK had low levels of resources and poor clinical outcomes, particularly in coronary heart disease and cancer survival (Berrino *et al.*, 1995) compared to other EU countries. In 2003, focusing on quality measures, Leatherman and Sutherland conducted what has been heralded as 'the most thorough review of data on quality [in the NHS] yet' (2003). They found a mixed picture of 'improvement, stasis and deterioration' (Leatherman and Sutherland, 2003). The number of patients waiting 12 months or longer for admission to hospital fell from 50 000 in 1999 to only 73 in late 2002, for example, but 20% of patients still wait more than six months and the number of operations cancelled at the last minute has risen. There are improvements to targets set in the National Service Frameworks (NSFs) but no data on conditions not covered by NSFs. The conclusion on the state of quality in the NHS, therefore, is one of cautious optimism. Further data and a longer period of time are needed before a more definite verdict can be advanced (Smith, 2003; Leatherman and Sutherland, 2003). A further report by Leatherman and Sutherland (2005) has been published coincidentally with this book.

Is the information we are collecting useful for evaluation?

Most health information systems were originally designed for financial management rather than evaluation purposes. Lack of available data may force healthcare systems to focus measurement on what is available, rather than what is most meaningful (Smith, 1995; Walshe, 2003). In the above example, NHS targets focused on the number of patients waiting more than 12 months for admission, without taking into account the growing number of patients whose surgeries are cancelled at the last minute (Smith, 2003). In this type of scenario, indicators may not necessarily reflect areas that need improvement, require prioritisation and match system goals (Smith, 1995; 2002; Walshe, 2003; Walshe and Freeman, 2002).

The culture of benchmarking has inadvertently led to a near-exclusive emphasis on the results of healthcare systems, with little attention to understanding why and how results have been obtained (Blalock, 1999). Lack of reliable data remains a significant impediment to any thorough evaluation of quality or performance within the NHS (Leatherman and Sutherland, 2003).

Is benchmarking guiding policy?

Although Marshall *et al.* (2003) suggest that the most important goal of benchmarking is to guide policy, several scholars have expressed fears that indicator measurement has become an end in itself. They have argued for the evaluation of benchmarking indicator systems and progression towards a true culture of performance (Blalock, 1999; Goddard *et al.*, 2000; Smith, 2002; Walshe, 2003). A House of Commons Public Administration Select Committee found that lack of articulation between policy objectives, targets and indicators undermined the credibility of benchmarking initiatives. It states:

> *Targets should never be accepted as a substitute for a clearly expressed strategy and set of priorities ... The target setting process has subverted this relationship with targets becoming almost an end in themselves, rather than providing an accurate measure of progress towards the organisation's goals and objectives. Targets can be good servants, but are poor masters.* (2003)

The fault does not lie with measurement efforts, but with the inadequate use and application of information produced. In political climates dominated by short-term imperatives and high media attention, there is inevitably a high risk of misinterpreting or misusing benchmarking data (Goddard *et al.*, 2000; McKee, 2002; Walshe *et al.*, 2001). Even when reliable evaluations do exist, findings are not necessarily translated into policy. Too few policies are evidence-based (Black, 2001; McIntyre *et al.*, 2001). These predictable weaknesses do not, however, make for a case against the benefits of benchmarking.

Improving benchmarking – the role of coherence, capacity and clinical engagement

Coherence, capacity and clinical engagement need to be emphasised to make current benchmarking more effective in driving healthcare system performance and quality (Smith, 2002).

'Coherence' implies that benchmarking initiatives fit in with other external review systems in place and that their roles are complementary and not duplicative or undermining. An example would be the efforts made to consolidate different 'arm's-length' bodies responsible for regulation and evaluation within the NHS. Consolidation is being evidenced in Scotland with the joining of different organisations under the umbrella of NHS Quality Improvement Scotland.

'Capacity' suggests that the healthcare system has the structures and skills in place to accommodate a performing benchmarking system and to ensure that it meets its objectives. It has implications for resources and cultural changes needed within healthcare systems at managerial and clinical levels.

Possibly the most critical success factor in benchmarking and evaluation efforts is 'clinical engagement'. A routine review and application of benchmarking data by clinical professionals is needed to improve data validity. This, in turn, will inform and improve clinical practice (Leatherman and Sutherland, 2003).

An audit of nine NHS hospital trusts found evidence of manipulation of waiting list data in order to meet government waiting list targets, often resulting in delayed treatment for other patients (Goddard *et al.*, 2000; NAO, 2001). 'Target fatigue' is a phrase coined to describe the lethargy brought on to hospitals, practitioners and local managers when faced with increasing checklists of targets and indicators but little rationale for how data will be used. In an evaluation of the impact of the Clinical Outcomes Indicators in Scotland, surveyed hospitals dismissed the information provided because of lack of credibility of the indicator framework, poor timeliness, little training and facilitation to interpret the data, no incentives to meet targets and no external accountability for the data (Goddard *et al.*, 2000). Clinical management needs to be matched with the engagement of executive management at all levels within the healthcare system.

To ensure useful, relevant benchmarking frameworks, the following aspects should be emphasised:

- *transparency* about the methods used to derive indicators and clear caveats about data limitations may help prevent inappropriate interpretation of results
- *a clear classification of target achievement*, such as the Scottish Executive's advocacy that targets be reported as 'achieved', 'ongoing', 'on track', 'delayed' or 'may not be achieved'
- *judicious selection of indicators and targets*
- *specification of the timeframe needed* to allow for meaningful interpretation
- *timeliness of data* to allow feedback to clinical practice
- *presentation of clusters of performance indicators* to avoid gaming and facilitate interpretation (Audit Commission, 2003).

Information, evaluation and benchmarking in joined-up policy

Greater emphasis on information, evaluation and benchmarking has implications for the other policy areas which will affect health and the healthcare system in years to come. Technology is fundamental to data collection and analysis. Other implications discussed here are in governance and care.

Although one of the stated objectives of benchmarking is to improve accountability across the healthcare system (Nutley and Smith, 1998), there is often a tension between centrally-driven performance management systems and decentralisation of service delivery and resource allocation. For this reason, policymakers have been advocating 'a new localism' in benchmarking (House of Commons Public Administration Select Committee, 2003) that combines clusters of national performance indicators with locally-set targets to foster improvement (Audit Commission, 2003; Scottish Executive, 2003). Further direct involvement of the public in setting policy goals and targets has been proposed but the willingness of the public to be involved in health policy making is questionable.

Similarly, although one of the stated aims of benchmarking is to allow individuals to make better choices about their care options (Nutley and Smith, 1998), there is evidence that the public do not use this information to guide treatment decisions (Marshall *et al.*, 2003). This may be due to lack of understanding of the data (Vaiana and McGlynn, 2002), limited trust in their provenance (Bentley and Nash, 1998) and no sense of ownership for the data produced. The question of who has responsibility within the system for conveying or translating this information to patients and their families needs to be considered.

However, still too little is known about whether the focus on data collection and benchmarking is actually contributing towards improving the health of our population (Sheldon, 1998). Most indicators reflect processes, not outcomes, of care (Goddard *et al.*, 2000). The 2004 Wanless report lamented the lack of evaluation data available to help guide future public health policies. The lack of a comprehensive evaluative framework for benchmarking makes it difficult to establish a causal relationship between specific processes of care and health outcomes. This precludes the possibility of making practical recommendations for meaningful service improvements (Nolte *et al.*, 2005) although early evidence of the use of indicators and targets in England would support their utility for improvement (Audit Commission, 2003).

Conclusions

These cross-cutting themes emerged from the process of undertaking the *Policy Futures for UK Health* project and the recognition of the difficulties associated with addressing health policy as a series of separate themes. Given the breadth and complexity associated with health policy, some sort of thematic focus is inevitable. The discussion of cross-cutting themes – a set of issues running through all the policy areas – demonstrates the strong need for policymakers to make connections across fields and to locate 'bits' of policy within a larger picture. On the one hand, this need to broaden thinking and joined-up policy is obvious. On the other, it has not yet been properly addressed. The preceding discussion of cross-cutting themes aims to point to where some important linkages may be, and thus to support more effective policymaking for the future.

References

Appleby J and Rosete AA (2003) The NHS: keeping up with the public expectations? In: A Parke, J Curtice, K Thomson, L Jarvis and C Bromley (eds) *British Social Attitudes: the 20th report – continuity and change over two decades.* Sage, London.

Association of Directors of Social Services (2000) *Prevention of Dependency in Older People.* Association of Directors of Social Services, London.

Astin JA (1998) Why patients use alternative medicine. *Journal of American Medical Administration.* 279: 1548–53.

Audit Commission (2003) *Targets in the Public Sector.* Audit Commission, London.

Barker DJP, Godfrey KM, Fall C, Osmond C, Winter PD and Shaheen SO (1991) Relation of birth weight and childhood respiratory infection to adult lung function and death from chronic obstructive airways disease. *British Medical Journal.* 303: 671–5.

Barnes R (2004) Glossary. http://www.who.int/hia/about/glos/en/. Accessed: 17 September 2004.

Bentley JM and Nash DB (1998) How Pennsylvania hospitals have responded to publicly released reports on coronary artery bypass graft surgery. *Joint Commission Journal on Quality Improvement.* 24(1): 40–9.

Berkman LF and Syme SL (1979) Social networks, host resistance, and mortality: a nine-year follow-up study of Alameda County residents. *American Journal of Epidemiology.* 109: 186–204.

Berrino F, Capocaccia R, Estève J, Gatta G, Hakulinen T, Micheli A, Sant M and Verdecchia A (1995) *Survival of Cancer Patients in Europe: the Eurocare study. No. 32.* International Agency for Research on Cancer, Lyon.

Best R (1995) The housing dimension. In: M Benzeval, K Judge and M Whitehead (eds) *Tackling Inequalities in Health – an agenda for action.* King's Fund, London.

Black N (2001) Evidence-based policy: proceed with care. *British Medical Journal.* 323(7307): 275–9.

Blalock AB (1999) Evaluation research and the performance management movement: from estrangement to useful integration? *Evaluation.* 5(2): 117–49.

Blum H (1981) *Planning for Health: genetics for the eighties.* Human Sciences Press, New York.

Brenner MH (1995) Political economy and health. In: BC Amick, S Levine, AR Tarlov and DC Walsh (eds) *Society and Health*. Oxford University Press, Oxford.

Britton A, Shipley M, Marmot M and Hemingway H (2004) Does access to cardiac investigation and treatment contribute to social and ethnic differences in coronary heart disease? Whitehall II prospective cohort study. *British Medical Journal*. **329**: 318.

Brocklehurst R and Costello J (2003) Health Inequalities: the Black Report and beyond. In: J Costello and M Haggard (eds) *Public Health and Society*. Palgrave Macmillan, Basingstoke, pp. 42–60.

Bunker J (2001) *Medicine Matters After All: measuring the benefits of medical care, a healthy lifestyle, and a just social environment*. The Nuffield Trust, London.

Cade JE, Barker DJP, Margretts BM and Morris JA (1988) Diet and inequalities in health in three English towns. *British Medical Journal*. **296**: 1359–62.

Cappuccio FP, Oakeshott P, Strazzullo P and Kerry SM (2002) Application of Framingham risk estimates to ethnic minorities in United Kingdom and implications for primary prevention of heart disease in general practice: cross sectional population based study. *British Medical Journal*. **325**: 1271.

Carr AJ, Gibson B and Robinson PG (2001) Measuring quality of life: is quality of life determined by expectations or experience? *British Medical Journal*. **322**: 1240–3.

City University London (2004) MSc economic evaluation in health care. Economic evaluation. Session 4. Equity. http://www.staff.city.ac.uk/~sm02571/eval4.doc. Accessed: 1 October 2004.

Coulter A (2002) *The Autonomous Patient: ending paternalism in medical care*. The Nuffield Trust, London.

Coulter A and Magee H (2003) *The European Patient of the Future*. McGraw Hill, Open University Press, Berkshire.

CPPIH (2004) *Commission for Patient and Public Involvement in Health website*. http://www.cppih.org/index.html. Accessed: 4 October 2004.

Dargie C (2000) *Policy Futures for UK Health. 2000 Report*. The Nuffield Trust, London.

Davey-Smith G, Hart C, Blane D, Gillis C and Hawthorne V (1997) Lifetime socio-economic position and mortality: perspective observational study. *British Medical Journal*. **314**: 547–52.

Dekkers F and Lister G (2002) *Self Care Lessons from Europe*. Department of Health Operations Research Department, Leeds.

DH (1997a) *The New NHS: modern, dependable*. Department of Health, London.

DH (1997b) *The NHS Plan: a first class service*. Department of Health, London.

DH (2000) *The NHS Plan: a plan for investment, a plan for reform. Cmnd 4818-I*. Department of Health, London.

DH (2004) *Choosing Health: making healthier choices easier. Cmnd 6374*. Department of Health, London.

DH (2005) *Independence, Well-being and Choice: our vision for the future of social care for adults in England: Social Care Green Paper. Cmnd 6499*. Department of Health, London.

DH and Social Services and Public Safety for Northern Ireland (2002) *Investing for health*. http://www.investingforhealthni.gov.uk/. Accessed: 27 March 2005.

Economic Policy Unit (2003) *Building on Progress: priorities for 2003–2004*. Department of Health, Belfast.

Evans RG and Stoddart GL (1990) Producing health, consuming health care. *Social Science & Medicine*. **31**(12): 1347–63.

Evans RG and Stoddart GL (1994) Producing health, consuming healthcare. In: RG Evans, ML Barer and TR Marmor (eds) *Why Are Some People Healthy and Others Not? The determinants of health of populations*. Walter de Gruyter, Berlin.

Farrell C (2004) *Patient and Public Involvement in Health: the evidence for policy implementation.* Department of Health, London.

Frank J, Ruggiero ED and Moloughney B (2003) *The Future of Public Health in Canada: developing a public health system for the 21st century.* Canadian Institutes of Health Research, Ottawa.

Gill PS, Kai J, Bhopal RS and Wild S. Black and minority ethnic groups. In: A Stevens *et al.* (eds) *Health Care Needs Assessment: the epidemiologically based needs assessment reviews. Third Series.* Radcliffe Publishing, Oxford. In press.

Glendinning C, Davies B, Pickard L and Comas-Herrera A (2004) *Funding Long-term Care for Older People: lessons from other countries.* Joseph Rowntree Foundation, York.

Goddard M, Mannion R and Smith P (2000) Enhancing performance in health care: a theoretical perspective on agency and the role of information. *Health Economics.* **9**: 95–107.

Hallqvist J, Lundberg M, Diderichsen F and Ahlbom A (1998) Socioeconomic differences in risk of myocardial infarction 1971–1994 in Sweden: time trends, relative risks and population attributable risks. *International Journal of Epidemiology.* **27**: 410–15.

Halpern D (1995) *Mental Health and the Built Environment.* Taylor & Francis, London.

Hamer L, Jacobson B, Flowers J and Johnstone F (2003) *Health Equity Audit Made Simple: a briefing for primary care trusts and local strategic partnerships working document.* Public Health Observatories, NHS Health Development Agency, London.

Health Information in Wales (2003) *Informing Healthcare: transforming healthcare using information and IT.* http://www.wales.nhs.uk/sites/documents/365/ihc-strategy-e.pdf. Accessed: 20 January 2005.

Hobbs M and Jamrozik K (2004) Medical care and public health. In: R Detels, J McEwen, R Beaglehole and H Tanaka (eds) *The Oxford Textbook on Public Health.* Oxford University Press, Oxford.

Holland W, Mossialos E, Belcher P and Merkel E (1998) *Public Health Decisions: methods of priority setting in the EU member states.* Office for Official Publications of the European Communities, Luxembourg.

House of Commons Public Administration Select Committee (2003) *On Target? Government by measurement. Fifth report of session 2002–2003.* The Stationery Office, London.

James WPT, Nelson M, Ralph A and Leather S (1997) The contribution of nutrition to inequalities in health. *British Medical Journal.* **314**: 1545–9.

Kirkwood T (2001) *The Reith Lectures 2001: The End of Age, Programme 5 – New Directions.* BBC, London.

Klein R (2003) Commentary: making policy in a fog. In: A Olivier and M Exworthy (eds) *Health Inequalities.* London School of Hygiene and Tropical Medicine, The Nuffield Trust, London.

Labonte R (1993) *Health Promotion and Empowerment: practice frameworks.* Center for Health Promotion and Participation, Toronto.

Lalonde M (1974) *A New Perspective on the Health of Canadians.* Ministry of National Health & Welfare, Ottawa.

Last J (1998) *Public Health and Human Ecology.* Appleton Lange, New York.

Leatherman S and Sutherland K (2003) *The Quest for Quality in the NHS: a mid-term evaluation of the ten-year quality agenda.* The Nuffield Trust, London.

Leatherman S and Sutherland K (2005) *The Quest for Quality in the NHS: a chartbook on quality of care in the UK.* Radcliffe Publishing, Oxford.

Lenaghan J (1998) *Brave New NHS? The impact of the new genetics on the health service.* Institute for Public Policy Research, London.

Lister G (2005) Health policy futures and cost scenarios for England 2003–2023. In: S Dawson and C Sausman (eds) *Future Health Organisations and Systems.* Palgrave Macmillan, Basingstoke.

Lowson K, West P, Chaplin S and O'Reilly J (2002) *Evaluation of Treating Patients Overseas: final report.* York Economics Consortium, York.

Macintyre S, McIver S and Sooman A (1993) Area, class and health: should we be focusing on people or places? *Journal of Social Policy.* **22**: 213–34.

Marmot M, Bobak M and Davy-Smith G (1995) Explanations for social inequalities in health. In: BC Amick, S Levine, AR Tarlov and DC Walsh (eds) *Society and Health.* Oxford University Press, Oxford.

Marshall MN, Shekelle PG, Davies HTO and Smith PC (2003) Public reporting on quality in the United States and the United Kingdom. *Health Affairs.* **22**(3): 134–48.

Mausner JS and Kramer S (1985) *Epidemiology: an introductory text.* WB Saunders Company, Philadelphia.

Maxwell R (1982) *Health and Wealth: international comparisons of health expenditure.* Simon and Schuster, New York.

McIntyre S, Chalmers I, Horton R and Smith R (2001) Using evidence to inform health policy: case study. *British Medical Journal.* **322**: 222–5.

McKee M (2002) Values, beliefs and implications. In: M Marinker (ed.) *Health Targets in Europe: polity, progress and promise.* BMJ Books, London.

McKeown T (1979) *The Role of Medicine.* Basil Blackwell, Oxford.

Millward LM, Kelly MP and Nutbeam D (2003) *Public Health Intervention Research: the evidence.* Health Development Agency, London.

Monaghan S, Huws D and Navarro M (2003) *The Case for a New UK Health of the People Act.* The Nuffield Trust, London.

Moore W (1999) The heart of the matter. *Health Matters.* www.healthmatters.co.uk.

Mossialos E (1997) *Citizens' Views on Health Care Systems in the 15 Member States: analysis of the Eurobarometer survey 1997.* Wiley Interscience, London.

NAO (2001) Tackling obesity in England. http://66.102.9.104/search?q=cache:H4htTWnvDHsJ: www.nao.org.uk/publications/nao_reports/00–01/0001220.pdf+Tackling+Obesity+in+England &hl=en&start=1&client=safari. Accessed: 16 March 2004.

Nolte E, McKee M and Wait S (2005) Describing and evaluating health systems. In: A Bowling and S Ebrahim (eds) *Handbook of Health Research Methods: investigation, measurement and analysis.* Open University Press, London.

Nutley S and Smith PC (1998) League tables for performance improvement in health care. *Journal of Health Services Research Policy.* **3**(1): 50–7.

ONS (2004) *Satisfaction with NHS GPs and Dentists: Social Trends 34.* Office of National Statistics, London.

Opinion Leader Research (2004) *Public Attitudes to Public Health Policy.* King's Fund, Health Development Agency, Department of Health, London.

Patrick DL and Wickizer TM (1995) Community and health. In: BC Amick, S Levine, AR Tarlov and DC Walsh (eds) *Society and Health.* Oxford University Press, Oxford.

Perfomance Assessment Network (2004) Quantitative indicators and published quality assessments – May 2004. http://www.paf.scot.nhs.uk/pafi/index.html. Accessed: 30 March 2005.

Rothstein B (2004) *The Universal Welfare State and Social Capital.* Fifth European Conference on Health Economics. London School of Economics, London.

Salomon JA, Tandon A and Murray CJL (2004) Comparability of self-rated health: cross-sectional multi-country survey using anchoring vignettes. *British Medical Journal.* **328**: 258–61.

Scottish Executive (2003) *NHS Scotland. Partnership for Care. Scotland's Health White Paper.* Scottish Executive, Edinburgh.

Secretary of State for Health (1999) *Saving Lives: our healthier nation. White Paper by the Secretary of State for Health*. Department of Health, London.

Sheldon T (1998) Promoting health care quality: what role performance indicators? *Quality in Health Care*. **7**: S45–50.

Smith J, Dame (2005) *The Shipman Inquiry – Fifth Report, Cmnd 6394-I, II, III. Safeguarding Patients: lessons from the past – proposals for the future*. The Stationery Office, London.

Smith PC (1995) On the unintended consequences of publishing performance data in the published sector. *International Journal of Public Administration*. **18**: 277–310.

Smith PC (2002) Performance management in British health care: will it deliver? *Health Affairs*. **21**(3): 103–15.

Smith R (2003) Is the NHS getting better or worse? We need better data to answer the question (editorial). *British Medical Journal*. **327**: 1239–41.

Social Services and Public Safety for Northern Ireland (2001) *The Future of Health Care and Care for the Elderly: guaranteeing accessibility, quality and financial viability*. European Commission.

Stratford N, Marteau T and Bobrow M (1999) Tailoring genes. In: R Jowell, J Curtice, A Park and K Thomson (eds) *British Social Attitudes, the 16th Report. Who Shares New Labour Values?* Ashgate Publishing, Aldershot, pp. 156–76.

The Royal Society and Royal Academy of Engineering (2003) *Nanotechnology: views of scientists and engineers*. The Royal Society, Royal Academy of Engineering, London.

Townsend P, Whitehead M and Davidson N (1992) *Inequalities in Health: the Black Report and the health divide*. Penguin Books, New York.

Turning Point (2004) Turning 40. http://www.turning-point.co.uk/NR/rdonlyres/64B6F401-3C9D-4853-AB88-5E6733090FCC/0/Turning40.pdf. Accessed: 4 October 2004.

Vaiana ME and McGlynn EA (2002) What cognitive science tells us about the design of reports for consumers. *Medical Care Research and Review*. **59**(1): 3–35.

Vallgarda S (2001) Governing people's lives. *European Journal of Public Health*. **11**(4): 386–92.

Vlad I (2003) Obesity costs UK economy £2bn a year. *British Medical Journal*. **327**: 1308.

Wait S (2004) *Benchmarking: a policy analysis*. The Nuffield Trust, London.

Wait S and Nolte E. Benchmarking health systems: trends, conceptual issues and future perspectives. *Benchmarking International Journal*. **12**(4/5). In press.

Walshe K (2003) International comparisons of the quality of health care: what do they tell us? *Quality and Safety in Health Care*. **12**: 4–5.

Walshe K and Freeman T (2002) Effectiveness of quality improvement: learning from evaluation. *Quality and Safety in Health Care*. **11**(1): 85–7.

Walshe K, Wallace L, Freeman T, Latham L and Spurgeon P (2001) The external review of quality improvement in health care organizations: a qualitative study. *International Journal of Quality Health Care*. **13**(5): 367–74.

Wanless D (2002) *Securing our Future Health: taking a long-term view*. HM Treasury, London.

Wanless D (2004) *Securing Good Health for the Whole Population. Final Report*. HM Treasury, London.

Wellcome Trust (2004) *Public Health Sciences: challenges and opportunities. Report of the Public Health Sciences Working Group convened by the Wellcome Trust*. The Wellcome Trust, London.

Whitehead M (1992) *The Concepts and Principles of Equity and Health*. World Health Organization, Copenhagen.

Whitehead M (1995) Tackling inequalities: a review of policy initiatives. In: M Benzeval, K Judge and M Whitehead (eds) *Tackling Inequalities in Health: an agenda for action*. King's Fund, London.

Wilkinson R (1997) Health inequalities: relative or absolute material standards. *British Medical Journal*. **314**: 591–5.

Wilkinson RG (1996) *Unhealthy Societies: the afflictions of inequality.* Routledge, London.

Wittenberg R, Hancock R, Comas-Herrera A and Pickard L (2002) Demand for long-term care in the UK: projections of long-term care finance for older people. In: R Brooks, S Regan and P Robinson (eds) *A New Contract for Retirement: modeling policy options to 2050.* Institute for Public Policy Research, London.

Zimmern RL and Cook C (2000) *The Nuffield Trust Genetics Scenario Project: genetics and health policy issues for genetic science and their implications for health and health services.* The Nuffield Trust, London.

Chapter 10

Future policy challenges

Sandra Dawson and Zoë Slote Morris

Each of the preceding chapters has given some view of the way in which UK health policy might develop in the future across the range of themes and concluded with recommendations specific to each chapter. This is a huge agenda including some major challenges. The foundation of the present is, however, strong. There have been many positive reforms to UK health policy since the publication of *Policy Futures for UK Health Report* in 2000, notably in increased funding, improved quality and a greater policy focus on health as opposed to healthcare.

However, this book has shown that serious policy issues remain for UK health in 2020. These emerged from different starting points, but are relevant to all the forgoing discussion. Five are highlighted here.

- There still needs to be stronger, more explicit, emphasis on health (including wellbeing) and an articulation of health as an individual entitlement and responsibility as well as a public good. To achieve greater clarity on this issue requires a review and restatement of the values underpinning health policy. This would have implications for entitlement, responsibilities and funding.
- A greater emphasis on health suggests that UK health policy must be located in wider social and economic policy contexts, as well as in a more global context.
- Government should review accountabilities within an increasingly fragmented health system. This places democratic, clinical and corporate governance at the centre of the policy agenda. It calls for a review of the purpose and scope of public and patient involvement in health policy and health, the public/private mix in funding and provision and the impact of devolution.
- In the context of explicitly-stated aims, purposes and responsibilities, government should provide strategic leadership for a more rational and planned system of health. This could involve stewardship by an independent body less vulnerable to election cycles and better able to work across sectors.
- An immediate and obvious challenge is the crisis in care. As demand increases and supply of both formal and informal care shrinks, new solutions need to be found, together with the money to pay for them. Self-care will undoubtedly be more significant but there remain outstanding questions about how this will be developed or sustained, and what it will imply for the hitherto important agendas of equity and access.

This book has outlined important factors shaping UK health policy to 2020. Some trends are clear; others are at a crossroads. Without doubt the future will see some renegotiation of the relationships between the state, the care professions and the individual, and also the nation state and other authorities.

Index